"*The CBT Workbook for Illness Anxiety* is an incredibly comprehensive resource that articulately explains everything you have ever wondered about illness anxiety or how to overcome it. Worden and Kaplan were able to share their deep knowledge of health anxiety and treatment in a manner that is equally informative yet digestible, and through a voice that is both supportive and kind. Unquestionably, this workbook will serve as a guiding light for so many who have struggled with illness anxiety by revealing the path back to a life that is no longer dictated by worries about health. This is a go-to book that I cannot wait to recommend to my clients and colleagues alike."

Alison R. Menatti, *Director, Center for OCD & Anxiety-Related Disorders, Saint Louis Behavioral Medicine Institute, MO*

"Drs. Kaplan and Worden have demonstrated exceptional proficiency in crafting a comprehensible and highly motivational text that adeptly elucidates the deleterious impacts of health anxiety and offers effective strategies for its mitigation. The inclusion of meticulously designed worksheets enhances the practical applicability of the content, while the periodic reinforcement of the underlying motivational principles adds a discernible level of efficacy to the overall therapeutic approach."

Mary E "Beth" Salcedo, *Medical Director, Ross Center, Washington, DC; past President of Anxiety and Depression Association of America*

The CBT Workbook for Illness Anxiety

This cognitive behavioral therapy (CBT) workbook is a detailed, step-by-step account of how to do scientifically supported treatment with adults experiencing illness anxiety.

Written by two practitioners with years of specialized training and expertise in CBT for anxiety, this book provides a comprehensive overview of illness anxiety disorder and an exposure-based framework to target fear and avoidance. Detailed exercises and homework are included throughout, as well as charts, diagrams, and a relapse prevention plan. This workbook aims to give illness anxiety sufferers the skills needed to work through the therapeutic journey in decreasing anxiety and beginning recovery.

This book is essential for those with illness- or health-related anxiety looking to do self-help or to use with therapists in sessions, along with practicing clinicians who need specialized guidance.

Blaise Worden is a clinical psychologist and researcher at the Institute of Living, Anxiety Disorders Center in Hartford, CT.

Johanna Kaplan is a clinical psychologist and director of the Washington Anxiety Center of Capitol Hill in Washington, DC.

The CBT Workbook for Illness Anxiety

Blaise Worden and Johanna Kaplan

Routledge
Taylor & Francis Group
NEW YORK AND LONDON

Designed cover image: Filmstax © Getty Images

First published 2025
by Routledge
605 Third Avenue, New York, NY 10158

and by Routledge
4 Park Square, Milton Park, Abingdon, Oxon, OX14 4RN

Routledge is an imprint of the Taylor & Francis Group, an informa business

© 2025 Blaise Worden and Johanna Kaplan

ISBN: 978-1-032-70733-4 (hbk)
ISBN: 978-1-032-71134-8 (pbk)
ISBN: 978-1-032-71135-5 (ebk)

DOI: 10.4324/9781032711355

Typeset in Palatino
by Deanta Global Publishing Services, Chennai, India

Contents

Acknowledgments . . . .*x*

1 Welcome to the Workbook 1
An Important Disclaimer about Medical Advice 3
Common Psychological Diagnoses Associated with
    Anxiety about Health 5
Finding Cognitive Behavioral Treatment for
    Illness-related Anxiety 16
Why You May Want to Consider Medication
    (Even Though You Probably Don't Want To) 18
Getting a Baseline Assessment of Your Illness Anxiety . . . 21
Health Anxiety Inventory (Short Version) 22
Motivation: Why Should I Take the Risk? 25

2 What Are My Problematic Health-related Beliefs? 38
What Are Your Illness Fears? 38
When You Are Anxious, You Are Not
    Thinking Clearly 46
Optional Exercise: Calculating the Estimated
    Probability of Your Scariest Scenario 58

3 What Are My Problematic Health-related Behaviors? 61
Potential Consequences of Excessive Health
    Information Seeking/avoidance 62
Health Behaviors Checklist 65
Gaining Awareness by Monitoring Anxious Responses 69
Anxiety Response Monitoring Form (Example) 70
Anxiety Response Monitoring Form 71
The Vicious Cycle of Anxious Behaviors 72

4 How Your Thinking Perpetuates Health Anxiety **75**
Common Health Myths 75
Doing a Cost-benefit Analysis of How Much Your
    Worry is Helping You............................. 94

5 Designing Your Exposure Hierarchy **98**
Approaching Health Fears........................... 98
Tips for Refining Your Exposure Hierarchy 115
Starting Exposures................................. 122

6 Common Cognitive Distortions **130**
Exposure Check-in and Troubleshooting.............. 130
Common Cognitive Distortions That Contribute to
    Anxiety 136
Common Cognitive Distortions in Health Anxiety 137
Practicing Talking Back to Your Anxious Thoughts..... 143
Thought-challenging Form (Example)................ 146
Thought-challenging Form 147

7 Interoceptive Exposures **148**
Check-in on Treatment Homework 148
Interoceptive Exposures............................ 153
Medical Readiness for Interoceptive Exposures........ 156
Doing Interoceptive Exposures 157
Core List of Interoceptive Exposures 158
Interoceptive Rating Form 167
My Interoceptive Exposure Practice Tracking Form 172
Some Additional Interoceptive Exposure Examples 176

8 Imaginal Exposures **179**
Check-in on Treatment Homework 179
Imaginal Exposures................................. 190
Sample Imaginal Exposures.......................... 195
Advanced Topic: Is Illness Anxiety Simply
    a Fear of Death?................................. 199
Religion, Spirituality, and Health Anxiety............. 204

9   **Giving Healthcare an Appropriate Role
    in Your Life** 207
    Check-in on Treatment Homework 207
    Moving Forward with Appropriate Health
       Behaviors 212

10 **Living a Life in Which Risk and Safety Are
    Balanced** 234
    Check-in on Treatment Homework and Progress 234
    Living a Valued Life and Accepting Anxiety........... 237
    Positive Preventative Health Behaviors and
       Adaptive Forms of Avoidance.................... 244

11 **Moving Forward and Embracing a Full Life.......... 248**
    Your Love–hate Relationship with Anxiety............ 248
    If I Am Not Living with My Health Anxiety,
       What Will I Spend My Time On? 250
    Relapse Prevention 254
    Health Anxiety Inventory (Short Version)............. 255
    Reaching Out to a Professional 265
    A Final (but Very Important) Note 266

References 269
Index 281

Acknowledgments

Much gratitude to our colleagues who have provided helpful feedback on this text, in particular Kimberly Sain, PhD, Eric WuLeung, MA, and Kelly Knowles, PhD, for their contributions. Many thanks to all the medical providers who provided commentary about their experience providing medical care to individuals with illness anxiety. Their names remain anonymous to ensure confidential, open comments, but their insights into medical practice in the context of illness anxiety are much appreciated! We are indebted to all the colleagues we work with each day who teach us their clinical expertise, share their research, and who have provided excellent ideas that we have integrated into either our clinical work or this text. We have learned much over the years from what you have shared about your compassionate, encouraging work with patients with illness anxiety. Finally, we'd like to express gratitude to the patients we work with every day who trust us with their care, who are brave enough to face their anxiety, and for their willingness to share their experiences with health-related anxiety so that others can learn from it.

For Dr. Kaplan:

"I would like to thank Tim, Ellie, and Tucker for their patience and allowing me space and time to dedicate to this important work. I would also like to thank Nancy Kaplan for her unending support and inspiration. Further, Dr. Worden has been a blessing and star in this book. I hope all who read this benefit greatly."

Crediting sources of third-party material using any wording requested with the grant of permission for use

Crediting third-party sources is not required as all text and graphic materials are self-created. References are appropriately cited. The questionnaire used in the text (Short Health Anxiety Inventory; SHAI) is open-source and appropriately cited.

1

Welcome to the Workbook

The two clinicians who collaborated to write this book are both specialists in the treatment and research of anxiety disorders. Together, we have decades of experience with treating illness anxiety (IA) and have treated hundreds of individuals with illness anxiety and related problems.

Psychologists have known for decades that cognitive behavioral therapy (CBT) for illness anxiety, as conducted by a trained therapist, has been shown to lead to notable reductions in symptoms of illness anxiety. Not only is it helpful, it is currently the most researched and most beneficial therapy for illness anxiety.[1] However, access to CBT for health-related anxiety can prove difficult, as qualified therapists can be hard to find. While this book is not meant to be a replacement for CBT with a skilled therapist, it is an excellent way to introduce yourself to the skills that are recommended to reduce illness anxiety. Most of the skills that we will recommend have been examined in various formats: one-on-one therapy, group therapy, internet-guided formats, and even self-help. We attempted to select skills that have been proven by science to be helpful when they are used regularly, and that have been the most helpful for our own patients. If you complete the book diligently, and practice all the exercises, you may find that your anxiety symptoms subside greatly. If not, later in the workbook we will talk about ways to find trained therapists and care providers who may be able to help you apply the skills and problem-solve potential barriers.

DOI: 10.4324/9781032711355-1

We are glad you are looking at this book to see if it might be helpful for your illness-related anxiety. Many people with anxiety about health attend many medical doctors' appointments, but may be reluctant to speak to a mental health expert about how psychological factors may contribute to their discomfort. It's not unusual for people to continue to present to medical doctors such as primary care providers, specialists, or at the emergency room, thinking that there must be medical explanations for their symptoms. In reality, psychological factors and medical factors are not separate things. The way that you think and behave (the psychological realm) impacts your health, physical sensations, how much pain and discomfort you experience, and vice versa. Therefore, it can help to step back and look at the whole picture. The brain and the body are connected in a multitude of complex ways.

You will see that we use the terms "illness anxiety" and "health anxiety" interchangeably throughout the course of the workbook. The term "illness anxiety" is generally used to denote a specific diagnosis that clinicians may give when anxiety about health reaches a certain level. In previous versions of our field's diagnostic manual, illness anxiety used to be referred to by the diagnostic label "hypochondriasis." That label is no longer formally used by clinicians, and most patients who have excessive health anxiety are diagnosed with either illness anxiety or a related issue, such as somatic symptom disorder or obsessive-compulsive disorder. Below, we will briefly discuss how clinicians might make a formal diagnosis of illness anxiety. However, anxiety about health is common even in healthy individuals, and can be thought of as being more on a spectrum, from adaptive and "normal" to not-so-adaptive and excessive. You do not need a formal diagnosis of illness anxiety to benefit from this book. If you are finding that your anxiety about health seems excessive to you or is causing you distress on a regular basis, you will likely find elements of this workbook to be helpful.

People may have worries about health for many different reasons. Just because you have worries that relate to health issues does not necessarily mean you have a clinical diagnosis. Illness anxiety is diagnosed when people have prolonged, excessive worry about the potential for developing or having a serious medical illness. However, worries about illness and things related to it are common with many other psychological disorders, and occur to some degree for most people. Below, we describe how illness anxiety is generally diagnosed, along with some brief descriptions of other diagnoses that are often quite like illness anxiety. While many of the strategies described in this workbook are helpful for many different anxiety issues, the skills that are recommended in the book are likely to be a best fit for illness anxiety. However, that does not mean that they cannot also be helpful for other conditions in which people may be excessively worried about health. It is possible to have more than one of the following diagnoses, and often these diagnoses are hard to differentiate because there is so much overlap in what the symptoms look like. If you are unsure which of the labels seems to apply to you, or whether this type of program may be most appropriate for you, you can always seek a professional clinician to obtain a formal evaluation and receive recommendations.

If you are following this workbook with the assistance of a therapist, it is designed so that it should roughly correspond to a chapter a week. Each week will typically involve a discussion of both behavioral and cognitive elements of treatment. However, it is more important that you give yourself time to digest and practice the material before proceeding to the next chapter. We therefore find that for most people in treatment, the workbook tends to take longer to progress through. Since the exercises tend to build on one another, we recommend you pace yourself accordingly. If you are using this workbook in conjunction with the therapist, bring it with you to the session. You want to make sure you are working on the same material at the same time. The quality of the patient–therapist relationship and effective communication one of the best predictors of a successful outcome in treatment.[2,3]

An Important Disclaimer about Medical Advice

Psychologists do not go to formal medical school to get their degree. While many of them have some degree of training and knowledge about some medical conditions and how they intersect with anxiety, psychologists are not formally qualified to provide medical advice. Therefore, nothing in this book will tell you directly when to see a doctor, what is a medical condition and what is not, when to be concerned about symptoms, and so on. When and how you choose to do exercises, and to what degree, will always be up to you. We consider this a very important part of treatment! Throughout the book we will discuss the importance of practicing tolerating uncertainty and learning to weigh information in unbiased ways in order to make your own conclusions about what is best for you, rather than letting anxiety make the decisions for you. We cannot tell you where to draw the line, we can only suggest what kinds of exercises have been shown to be beneficial based on the scientific research, and examples of some things that have worked for our patients.

That said, everyone is different and has a different body with different symptoms, contexts, and different values. We respect your ability to choose what you think is best for yourself and your body, and therefore will never tell you what to do with it! Some people will need to alter exercises described in the book based on ongoing medical conditions, and one size does not fit all.

You may find this lack of direct reassurance frustrating. Most people with illness anxiety (and anxiety disorders in general) prefer certainty. They tend to go out of their way to try and get more certainty, often to the point that it backfires for them as they become preoccupied with rare possibilities. Therefore, hearing that you will not get concrete answers about your health from this book may sound disappointing! What we can tell you is that practicing tolerating such uncertainty is ideal, and that decades of scientific research has supported walking towards your fears (exposure therapy) as the gold-standard method of treating a variety of anxiety issues.

Given that individuals with illness anxiety tend to report more physical signs and symptoms than non-health-anxious people, and that anxiety issues can sometimes be caused or maintained by medical factors, we typically recommend that prior to starting this program you are evaluated by medical professionals to rule out or examine medical explanations for symptoms. However, once you have shared your concerns with your medical practitioner, it is important to be extremely judicious about continued medical visits. Feel free to discuss your medical concerns with your therapist, and if necessary, they may advise medical consultation before you take a step forward (e.g., seeking out additional medical assessment or continuing to work through the health anxiety). Working in concert with a medical provider is key to be able to untangle a complicated diagnostic differential.

That said, the presence of actual medical conditions or symptoms does not prohibit treatment for illness anxiety. As mentioned above, we expect most individuals with health-related anxiety to notice more signs and symptoms. Many of our referrals come from medical professionals who have told their anxious patients to seek psychological treatment! We tend to proceed with treatment if participants agree that their level of anxiety about health seems excessive to them—that is, beyond what they think is reasonable for someone with that medical issue or symptom(s).

Common Psychological Diagnoses Associated with Anxiety about Health

Mental health professionals use a guide called the *Diagnostic and Statistical Manual of Psychological Disorders* (DSM-5)[4] to assist in diagnosis of specific psychological issues. The diagnoses in this manual have been developed by workgroups of experts that are tasked with integrating all the known information about mental health symptoms to make meaningful categories and diagnostic labels. Mental disorders are not like many medical disorders, in that they cannot be identified based on tests that screen for the presence of a certain bacteria, gene, or other physical indicator. Instead, psychological diagnoses are typically based on the self-report of the person experiencing the symptoms. Therefore, in some ways the experience of anxiety is subjective. However, this does not mean that the symptoms are not "real." Take a more medically familiar variable, such as pain. Pain is also subjective. When a patient goes to the emergency room, patients are often asked to use a chart to rate their pain on a scale of 0–10. Pain is a subjective as well, but a valid experience, like anxiety.

Below we describe several clinical mental health diagnoses/ conditions that have been typically associated with anxiety about health-related issues. In our opinion, it is less important to decide on the appropriate label, as long as in reading the description of this treatment you think this treatment will be helpful for you.

Illness Anxiety (a.k.a. "Health Anxiety" or Hypochondriasis)

People with illness anxiety worry excessively about potentially having or developing a serious medical condition. The worry about health occurs on a daily or near-daily basis. However, many patients report that when they are not having active physical symptoms, they tend to not catastrophize as much.

In illness anxiety, fear about health tends to be disproportionate to the actual risk of a serious medical condition. A patient may have spoken with doctors who have reassured them about their symptoms, although this may have led to only brief relief before worry and anxiety reemerged. Another possibility is that they may have no symptoms at all, and simply worry about the potential of developing signs of serious illness.

When weird new bodily sensations arise, as is quite normal and expected as we age, individuals with IA are likely to interpret them as signs that there is something seriously medically wrong with them.[5] Some illness-anxious patients have expectations that their subjective experience of their health should not change as they naturally age and therefore are quite concerned when natural changes do occur. They are often engaging in many behaviors designed to give them a sense of control over their health. Some individuals will engage in reassurance behaviors, such as seeing doctors excessively, researching medical symptoms on the internet, asking for reassurance from friends or family members, or checking their body for signs of illness. Others with illness anxiety will prefer to avoid health cues (e.g., avoiding doctor's visits for fear that they will get bad news or discover signs of illness). These behaviors are called safety behaviors. They are designed to give you a sense of control over health. Such safety behaviors tend to backfire in the long run, in that they prevent you from learning that health fears may not be accurate, and prevent you from learning that you do not need to rely on these behaviors for anxiety to go away and for your physical health to be maintained. Even as fears are quelled, either by avoidance or excessive reinforcement in doctor visits, new health fears replace old ones and the health anxiety cycle continues to flourish.

Illness anxiety is very common, with estimates of around 2 to 4.5% of the population meeting criteria for a full diagnosis.[6] That means that in any given crowd of 100 people, at least two people will likely have significant illness anxiety! Many more people likely have *subclinical* anxiety about health—that is, anxiety about health that is strong but that may not impair functioning or cause significant distress. Despite being classified as a somatoform disorder (and not an anxiety disorder) in the *Diagnostic and Statistical Manual* (DSM-5) that psychologists use to diagnose, many researchers have argued that illness anxiety is more closely related to OCD and anxiety disorders. The protocol that we outline in this book for the treatment of illness anxiety is rooted in cognitive behavioral treatment of anxiety disorders.

Obsessive-compulsive Disorder

Differentiating illness anxiety from OCD may be difficult and is not always clear-cut, as the disorders can have a lot of symptom overlap. Health concerns, especially those surrounding fears of contamination (i.e., getting ill from the spread of germs or viruses) are very common concerns in OCD. Both individuals with IA and individuals with health or contamination-related OCD may worry excessively that they are going to develop or already have a serious medical illness. Both also are likely to show excessive health behaviors—things that people may do to control their health or get more certainty about health. Compulsions are typically a major component of OCD. Compulsions are behaviors that people complete (either overtly or covertly) to try and reduce anxiety associated with obsessions, or to get more certainty. Therefore, compulsions often look very similar to health-related behaviors that people do in illness anxiety. In reality, they are often very difficult to differentiate, and even trained professionals struggle with this.

One potential factor that may help discriminate between diagnoses is the nature of the anxious thoughts. Individuals with OCD tend to have obsessional thoughts or urgers that are "not-me" thoughts—psychologists often call these "ego-dystonic" thoughts. These are thoughts, urges, or strong feelings that people may feel but not necessarily agree with, which leads to that feeling of being compelled. For individuals with OCD, there is a disconnect between the "feeling" parts of the decision-making brain and the "thinking" parts. This leads to the feelings brain sending strong messages that something is wrong, while the thinking brain is still intact and may simultaneously know that the facts do not seem to match up to the feelings. What that means is that individuals with OCD often have a strong emotional feeling that an outcome will occur, but often when pinned down are typically able to recognize that fears are highly excessive. They may also be likely to recognize, at least at times, that compulsions can have a magical quality to them—that is, they are not realistically likely to reduce risk. For example, a person with OCD may feel that if they stomp their feet 20 times, they will not get a disease that day. This person is likely able to recognize at least in part that stomping their feet is not directly related to health, but still feels compelled to complete this action as it is temporarily relieving. Individuals with IA are more likely to believe that their feared health outcomes are realistic and that the behaviors they are doing to mitigate these outcomes are helping in some way. Why is this distinction important? Because current treatment for OCD focuses on recognizing that the "feelings" brain is like a loud alarm, but just because an alarm is loud does not necessarily mean that it is correct. You can use your thinking brain instead, to step back from the loud alarm and look at facts and figures to determine the best course of action without engaging in compulsions. The core of the treatment is awareness of this discrepancy. In illness anxiety, there may be some discrepancy, but often less so. Therefore, a person with illness anxiety may not initially believe that their health-related behaviors are excessive. In this way, illness anxiety can be similar to forms of OCD with limited insight. Because certainty is often so strong, trying to refrain from health behaviors is often hard in the beginning, as it feels so risky. Therefore, some examination and challenging of anxious thoughts is often very appropriate for individuals with illness anxiety prior to testing out some of these beliefs with exposures. Often in OCD, cognitive challenging is not necessary and exposure work can be completed immediately.

Finally, in discriminating OCD from illness anxiety, fears in OCD are often contamination-related and therefore tend to be more likely to be communicable diseases. Fears in illness anxiety tend to be severe, uncommunicable diseases,[5] such as cancer, strokes, heart disease, or Lou Gherig's disease. While there are certainly exceptions to this, considering the nature of the fears can help differentiate when you ares on the fence. In fact, OCD and illness anxiety co-occur relatively commonly,[7][8] and health-related concerns, particularly fears of contamination, are one of the most common themes of OCD.[9]

An example of OCD may be *John*, who worries constantly that he may get COVID. He has been avoiding interacting with others aside from his three coworkers, who he knows are vaccinated. He asks them daily if they have been in contact with anyone who is ill. Every time he enters his home, he must wash for at least two minutes, using at least three pumps of soap. Any time he notices a physical symptom, he immediately starts to worry that he has COVID and tries to arrange for a diagnostic test as soon as possible. He researches the latest information about the virus statistics daily, and researches about what precautions to take. From all his reading and research on the virus, he is aware that his precautions are highly excessive, and that many of them are statistically unlikely to reduce his risk, stating "I know what I am doing is irrational, but I still feel I have to do it."

Another example of OCD would be *David*, who fears that he must shave his head and keep it very clean in case he gets an ingrown hair, which can cause an infection, which will go to his brain and cause death. He spends hours every night cleaning his head, shaving it, and using tweezers to pull out any hairs he suspects may be ingrown or cause infection. David has never experienced an ingrown hair, but reported hearing stories from friends of how painful they were and how they can cause a whole-body infection. He states that while he knows his behaviors are excessive, he feels compelled to engage in them for fear he may get such an infection.

Somatic Symptom Disorder

Somatic Symptom Disorder is another diagnosis that is very similar to illness anxiety and has a lot of overlap. In fact, they are so similar, some researchers have suggested that illness anxiety and somatic symptom disorder may not actually be different disorders, but rather related problems on a spectrum of health-related anxiety.[10, 11] The primary difference is that people with somatic symptom disorder are often overly concerned about reducing the discomfort and impairment related to existing physical symptoms or conditions, while people with illness anxiety are generally concerned about the potential of developing a serious issue and are therefore concerned about what the symptoms might *mean*. Individuals with illness anxiety also may experience intermittent uncomfortable physical symptoms and conditions that lead them to feel excessively anxious about the impact of the symptoms, but typically these symptoms are intermittent and not occurring on a daily or near-daily basis, as they do in somatic symptom disorder.

Individuals with somatic symptom disorder tend to have chronic physical symptoms, and these symptoms may even be related to an established medical issue, but these individuals tend to be overly preoccupied with their medical symptoms, overcautious, and excessively avoiding activities due to fears of worsening medical symptoms. Like individuals with illness anxiety, individuals with somatic symptom disorder may also worry that their physical symptoms are signs of serious medical issues, despite a lack of concrete evidence.

It is appropriate to have some level of concern, worry, and discomfort related to many medical conditions; however, those with somatic symptom disorder tend to worry about the impact of their medical conditions and physical symptoms more than would be considered clinically appropriate. Oftentimes, they are refraining from engaging in activities or otherwise overprotecting themselves to not make symptoms worse, even when a physician has not explicitly directed them to do these things. They also misinterpret discussions with their physicians (e.g., the discussion of having high cholesterol in your family as a sign that they in fact will develop it almost immediately). They worry daily about their medical symptoms, and the worry is disproportionate to the scale of the actual symptoms/medical issue.

An example of someone who has somatic symptom disorder may be *Maria*, who has long experienced physical symptoms such as recurrent migraine headaches, back and neck pain, and a variety of forms of stomach discomfort. While her doctors have not found any medical diagnoses to explain most of her symptoms, they recently informed her she likely has developed irritable bowel syndrome (IBS). Maria worries daily about the potential for worsening her physical symptoms and is avoiding certain activities—e.g., exercising, spicy foods, moving her head too quickly—as she fears that they will worsen her physical symptoms. Certainly, conditions such as IBS often lead to some physical discomfort and may require some adaptations to life to manage and minimize the interference. For example, Maria's doctor recommended that certain types of acidic foods are generally best avoided, supplements are taken, efforts are made to stay hydrated, and strenuous activities are paced. However, Maria reads into this advice and engages in more protective behaviors than are helpful, such as limiting most of her activities outside the home, refusing to go places where she does not have easy access to the bathroom, lying down whenever she feels the slightest bit of physical discomfort, and refusing to eat any foods that she suspects have ever led to an increase in discomfort. She worries about the medical condition and its implications for hours daily, despite her doctor informing her that IBS is a manageable condition and can be treated, and does not need to strongly inhibit life in most cases. She believes she is an exception to the doctor's rule (i.e., she is a special case and her life will be severely disrupted).

Panic Disorder

Individuals with panic disorder (PD) are primarily worried about having panic attacks, which are sudden, relatively brief "attacks" of at least four of the following symptoms happening at once and hitting a peak within 10–15 minutes: heart racing, dizziness, excessive sweating, choking feelings, chest pressure, vision blurring, stomach upset, difficulty/pressure breathing, feelings of going crazy or losing control, fear of dying, feelings of tingling or numbness in your extremities. Just having had some panic attacks does not mean that you have panic disorder, as panic attacks can happen alongside many disorders. To get the diagnosis of panic disorder, you must be worried about panic attacks that seem to come on out of the blue, rather than caused by something that you are doing or worrying about. People with panic disorder fear when and where they will have a panic attack, and about what the panic attack might mean—for example worrying that they may go crazy, lose control, pass out, or have a heart attack and die. Because of this, panic disorder can seem very similar to heath anxiety, because a person may have fears that their physical panic attack symptoms may be signs of an underlying medical problem such as a heart attack or stroke. However, individuals with PD are mostly worried about the consequences of the panic attacks themselves, and report that if the panic attacks would magically disappear, they would not have a problem anymore. They tend to not worry about medical issues outside of the panic episodes, and do not engage in the frequency of heath-checking behaviors that are associated with illness anxiety. In addition, panic disorder is frequently co-diagnosed with agoraphobia, which is when people are avoiding or having difficulty tolerating situations in which they are worried they may not be able to escape or get help in the case of sudden panic symptoms. Often these situations are places like elevators, crowds, being far from home, airplanes, etc., as these are settings in which people can often feel trapped and have some concern about being able to get out or get assistance if they have a sudden panic attack.

An example of panic disorder may be *Timothy*, who reports having around one panic attack per day. He reports that these attacks seem to come on out of the blue, and consist of suddenly feeling very dizzy, lightheaded, feeling "dreamlike," heart racing, and having difficulty swallowing. He reports that when these attacks occur, he worries intensely that he will faint, even though he has never fainted in his life. He also has some worry that the dizziness and dreamlike feeling is a sign that he may be having a stroke or indicators, despite his having a lack of notable risk factors for these sudden medical problems.

Generalized Anxiety Disorder

Generalized anxiety disorder (GAD) is a disorder characterized by daily, excessive worry. Some prominent psychologists were considering changing the name of GAD to "excessive worry disorder" because that's exactly what it is—excessive worry. People with GAD tend to worry about the same things as others, but find the worry harder to control, and worry so often each day that it is causing some wear and tear on the body, such as lack of sleep, chronic muscle and emotional tension, difficulty concentrating, and irritability. It's not unusual for individuals with GAD to have physical symptoms that are likely a result of prolonged worry and anxiety: indigestion, nausea, or diarrhea, headaches, and muscle tension. GAD can be difficult to differentiate from illness anxiety, as a common worry domain in GAD is related to health and health of family members. One defining feature in GAD is that the excessive worries are present across several different events or activities (i.e., more than one domain of worry). Further, the domain of worry will likely shift from one topic to another over time. Thus, examining if someone worries about multiple domains in life or solely health-related topics is often a helpful diagnostic distinction. In GAD, the tendency to over-fret is the problem, and the content of the worry tends to be just a foil for an excessive problem-solving and ruminative-thinking style. Patients with GAD often report a sense that if one issue they were worrying about were to be resolved, that would be replaced with another concern/worry.

An example of GAD may be *Janet*. Janet worries that their occasional physical symptoms are signs of serious illness. Unlike individuals with a diagnosis of illness anxiety, however, Janet only occasionally worries excessively about their health, and in addition to health, worries frequently about several other things, such as whether their adult son will be able to lose weight, whether they will have enough money to retire, and whether they are good enough at their job. They report that their worry is keeping them up at night. Janet often feels irritable and snaps at family and friends, and has frequent headaches and feels tired from chronic tension.

Posttraumatic Stress Disorder

One final diagnosis we will mention as one that might be conflated with illness anxiety is posttraumatic stress disorder (PTSD). PTSD can occur when someone has been through a traumatic experience: an experience in which they thought they might die or be seriously harmed, or witnessed extreme violence. In some cases, someone has been through a very traumatic medical experience for which they may have posttraumatic symptoms, although typically the medical issue onset is sudden, life-threatening, and the person experiences intense fear for their life or safety. The difference between PTSD and some of the other disorders mentioned above is that PTSD is typically not limited to just fears about illness. It tends to come with other symptoms, such as nightmares or flashbacks about the traumatic event, hypervigilance, feeling jumpy or startling easily, and feeling very irritable. Individuals with PTSD often avoid try to avoid thinking or talking about their trauma, and tend to be avoiding some cues that remind them of the traumatic event, such as people, places, sounds, or smells that were associated with it. Most people with PTSD report that the traumatic event has changed how they view themselves or the world. For example, they may have developed beliefs such as "people are not trustworthy," "one must always look out for danger," "things I care about can be taken away at any minute," and so on. They may feel excessively guilty, or feel like they are disconnected from intimate emotional connections with others.

One example of an individual with PTSD is *Frank*. He had an unexplained serious medical event that resulted in a procedure in which he was told he would not survive. He was awake but restrained during the procedure, and recalls feeling terrified. While Frank survived the ordeal and has a good prognosis now, he continues to feel highly anxious and apprehensive, despite having limited anxiety about health prior to the event. He becomes tearful whenever someone brings up a serious procedure that they went through, and refuses to talk about the medical event with friends or family. Since the traumatic event, he has difficulty being in or around medical centers, talking to doctors, or smelling sterilizing agents. He says that he continues to have nightmares and unwanted flashbacks to being restrained in the hospital fearing that he would die. He now has great mistrust of medical providers, and greatly fears developing an illness that will lead him to have to interact with a medical provider.

Appropriate Health-related Concern or Adjustment to a Health Condition

A final domain to consider is appropriate concern about health issues. Medical conditions, especially those that lead to chronic disability or pain, are expected to lead to some distress, and we would consider this expected and not necessarily pathological. Not all health-related anxiety is problematic or a diagnosable issue that warrants treatment. Usually, formal psychological diagnoses are made when the anxiety is either excessively distressing to the person, or significantly impairing their daily functioning (e.g., they are avoiding situations they may not need to avoid because of anxiety).

Some people may experience a significant increase in anxiety when they are trying to adjust to a new diagnosis of a medical condition, or when they are having difficulty coping with an ongoing chronic medical illness. There are perfectly normal emotional responses to the difficulties associated with medical conditions, which may include feeling grief for the loss of some independence, feeling frustrated with pain or interference, or feeling unsure about what are the best guidelines for managing the condition. If you are experiencing distressing health-related anxiety, but feel it is proportionate to the health-related stressors you are facing, you may want to consider seeing a health psychologist. A health psychologist is a psychologist who is knowledgeable about several health conditions and who can help provide guidance on how to manage or reduce the psychological burden of health issues. They often work on improving physical health by improving mental health. They do a variety of things, but may do things such as educate about how behavioral changes can make a difference in diabetes care, help people find cancer support groups, help a patient outline a specific plan to reduce emotional eating for weight loss to prevent worsening of heart disease, and may even do cognitive behavioral treatment for issues such a chronic pain or insomnia.

Parsing these things out can be difficult, so if you are unsure, we encourage you to seek an evaluation with a mental health professional who will likely be able to make recommendations about what kind of mental health assistance may be necessary.

Finding Cognitive Behavioral Treatment for Illness-related Anxiety

This workbook is based on a cognitive behavioral treatment model, and uses the same principles that cognitive behavioral psychologists use in treating their patients with illness anxiety. We use CBT as it is currently the gold-standard, most effective psychological treatment for nearly all fear-based disorders.[12–16] CBT is a broad framework for understanding treatment and mental health, and discussing the full theory behind it is beyond the scope of this book. In short, however, it involves talking about your cognitions, or how you think, and your behaviors, and how they may be maintaining anxiety in your current life. Cognitions-wise, when people are anxious, they tend to think in ways that inadvertently maintain their anxiety. They also engage in behaviors that while well-intentioned, tend to maintain anxiety problems. CBT aims to help people identify these not-so-helpful patterns and change them so that the cycle of anxiety does not get perpetuated.

Although CBT has been shown to be quite effective in terms of reducing illness anxiety symptoms for many people, it's not a cure-all. Most people with illness anxiety who complete a course of CBT treatment with a therapist will show reductions in symptoms of about 19–29% at the end of treatment,[1] which usually involves once-weekly sessions over several months. About half of the people who do CBT for illness anxiety are considered in remission after a course of treatment.[17] What that means is that their scores on measures of illness anxiety after treatment are closer to individuals who don't have a diagnosis than to individuals who do. Most people have also been shown to maintain these gains at follow-up more than a year later.[1] At least one study[18] suggests that bibliotherapy (or reading a book on how to treat illness anxiety, such as this one!) is also an effective treatment for illness anxiety. However, for the treatment to work maximally, it likely must involve exposure,[18, 19] which just means practice in gradually confronting your fears. As we believe this is the most important part of tackling anxiety, we will explain a lot more about exposures in this book.

A small number of other psychological (non-medication) treatments have been examined to see how effective they are in treating illness anxiety. However, there is currently only a small amount of research on these treatments, and it remains unclear how well they may work for illness anxiety-related concerns and whether they are effective in the long term.

This workbook is not intended to be a substitute for skilled care with a clinician who is knowledgeable about illness anxiety. If you are having difficulty implementing the techniques in the book or feel unsure if the book is appropriate for you, you may want to try to connect with a licensed therapist who can provide further assessment and guidance. Some clinicians may also use this book as a workbook throughout the course of treatment. The most useful way to proceed through this book is giving yourself enough time, space, and social support to digest it thoroughly.

We know that finding a therapist who is knowledgeable about illness anxiety can be very difficult. It is likely easiest to start with searching for therapists who are trained in CBT for anxiety disorders or obsessive-compulsive and related disorders. There is a US national organization for providers who are trained in CBT, called the Association for Behavioral and Cognitive Therapies. Its website, ABCT.org, has a find-a-therapist directory that can be searched by region and specialty. This is an excellent place to start, although not all providers may have training or expertise in illness anxiety specifically. Another organization that may be helpful is the International Obsessive-Compulsive Foundation, currently at IOCDF.org. It also has a directory with a listing of therapists who specialize in OCD-related disorders. This may be a good option if your anxiety about health is related to OCD.

Why You May Want to Consider Medication (Even Though You Probably Don't Want To)

Most people with illness anxiety prefer non-medication treatments, such as CBT. Because you are anxious about health, the prospect of taking new medications, or taking medications at all, might feel daunting. Many people are worried about the side effects that come along with medications, or worried about long-term effects of taking medications. However, we believe medications can be helpful in reducing illness anxiety for many people.

We should remind you here that the authors of this book are psychologists, not psychiatrists. What that means is that we are specialists in psychological therapy, rather than medications. We are not prescribers, and do not have the necessary requirements to do so, such as medical school training. Therefore, the comments about medications below are generalities, and if you have any questions about medications or other biological options, please speak with a prescriber, such as a doctor of medicine or advanced practice registered nurse (APRN) who can provide you with more details!

There aren't currently any medications that are specifically indicated for the treatment of illness anxiety. However, there are decades of research on medication treatments for anxiety disorders that may be informative. There have also been a few studies specifically examining the usefulness of medications in treating illness anxiety. This research suggests that some medications, those that are commonly prescribed for anxiety disorders or depression, may be helpful for some people in reducing symptoms of illness anxiety.[17, 20–22] These medications tend to be in the class of medications called "antidepressants." Around 30–60% of people report noticeable reductions in anxiety symptoms with these medications.[17, 21, 23] These medications have been used for decades to treat depression and anxiety, and currently are recommended by many reputable international medical organizations as the frontline medical option for most anxiety issues.[24-27] Specifically, these medications are a type of antidepressant called SSRIs, which stands for selective serotonin reuptake inhibitors, or SNRIs, serotonin and norepinephrine reuptake inhibitors. These medications work on how brain chemicals such as serotonin are processed in the brain. The brain chemicals that are impacted are part of human brain functioning and therefore already in your brain—the medications just help your brain access them better. These medications will not change your personality. They also won't suddenly make you an overly positive, anxiety-free person. In addition, people with illness anxiety often have co-occurring issues, like depression or other anxiety disorders, and these medications can also help target those symptoms, which may indirectly improve anxiety about health. While medications may be helpful on their own, there is some evidence to suggest that people are more likely to relapse to anxiety issues when they discontinue the medications if they have not completed CBT. Therefore, when it comes to anxiety issues, we normally suggest people consider CBT in combination with antidepressant medications, as the highest success rates tend to occur when people do both: they take medications *and* engage in CBT.[28-30]

There is another class of medication that is commonly prescribed for anxiety disorders, and that is the class of medications called benzodiazepines. Benzodiazepines are a type of sedative, and work differently than the antidepressant class of medications. They have some potential for misuse and addiction if they are overused.[31] Therefore, it's typically not recommended for them to be taken in high or frequent doses or to be taken for long periods of time.[32] While antidepressants are prescribed to be taken on a daily basis, benzodiazepines are often prescribed on a pro re neta, or as-needed, basis, to be taken in cases of extreme anxiety. Benzodiazepine medications are certainly commonly prescribed for anxiety disorders,[33] likely as much or more than antidepressants.[34] In addition, patients taking them often report that they are effective at reducing anxiety in the moment, and that they tend to work as well in the short term at managing anxiety as the antidepressant class of medications. However, many cognitive behavioral psychologists have expressed some reservations about the use of benzodiazepine medications, especially when they are taken only in response to strong anxiety. Why might this be a problem? The argument is that taking the medication in response to anxiety is a protective behavior that prevents people from learning that they do not need the medication to survive the situation. If someone is particularly afraid of feeling anxious, this will lower their ability to see that they can tolerate anxiety, and that without protective responses, it will always go away in time. We will talk much more in the book about why this approach of tolerating anxiety and approaching fears is helpful. But in short, the sedative medications may be more likely to interfere with exposure-based treatment, making it less likely that people benefit. There is some evidence to suggest this may be the case, with individuals who take benzodiazepines on an as-needed basis showing somewhat less response to CBT.[35, 36]

Because people with illness anxiety are hyper-aware of bodily symptoms and easily alarmed by them, starting new medications is usually more difficult than it may be for others. Chances are, because you are worried about physical symptoms, you will be more likely to notice minor side effects and catastrophize about them—worrying that they will last forever, will create some sort of lasting damage, or that they are signs of something more serious. Individuals with illness anxiety are also more likely to notice any side effects, as they are particularly good at scanning their body for signs of disruption. However, that means they will notice more and fret about things that are likely benign symptoms that others tolerate. Medication side effects can often be strongest when a medication is started, leading many anxious people to start and then abruptly discontinue a medication, never allowing it to get up to its full helping potential. However, if you are able to tolerate some discomfort and uncertainty that might arise, there is a good chance that medications might be helpful in the long run.

Even if you have tried some psychiatric medications in the past and found them not so helpful, it may be worth meeting with a psychiatrist or psychiatric APRN who may be able to reevaluate your symptoms and give a second opinion. There are many different medications, and it is unfortunately not unusual for people to have to try several before they find one that seems to "click" for their personal biology. In addition, medication research and development change rapidly, so if it has been a while since you have spoken with a prescriber about your anxiety, you may want to talk with them about newer medications that may be a better match or that may have lower side effect profiles for you. If you have a specific side effect that you are particularly concerned about and feel will be a serious no-go for you, keep in mind that there are many medications, and prescribers may be able to minimize or avoid certain side effects. In addition, don't forget that you can always listen to what the prescriber has to say and then decide whether to take the medications or not after you hear about potential side effects or other consequences. Just because you meet with a prescriber does not mean that you must commit to taking medications. For many people, side effects are limited, and for many people the reduction that they find in their anxiety about health may be worth it. In addition, later in this book we will encourage you to practice tolerating normal physical sensations. Therefore, the experience of some mild side effects is often an excellent opportunity to practice tolerating sensations.

Getting a Baseline Assessment of Your Illness Anxiety

When we are working on any aspect of mental health, it can be hard to tell if we are making progress over time. Change can be gradual and slow, so we might not realize change over time, or remember how things were before we started to work on our problems. Below is the Short Health Anxiety Inventory, developed by Salkovskis and colleagues,[37] to help you assess your current level of anxiety about health. Once you have completed the workbook, you can also re-administer it to see if you have had a reduction in your total score, so you may want to save your responses for comparison later.

Health Anxiety Inventory (Short Version)[37]

. Each question in this section consists of four statements. Please read each group of statements carefully, and then select the one which best describes your feelings over the past six months. Identify the statement by circling the letter next to it—i.e. if you think that statement (a) is correct, circle statement (a); it may be that more than one statement applies, in which case, please circle any that are applicable.

---

1.   (a) I do not worry about my health
      (b) I occasionally worry about my health
      (c) I spend much of my time worrying about my health
      (d) I spend most of my time worrying about my health

2.   (a) I notice aches/pains less than most other people (of my age)
      (b) I notice aches/pain a much as most other people (of my age)
      (c) I notice aches/pains more than most other people (of my age)
      (d) I am aware of aches/pains in my body all the time

3.   (a) As a rule I am not aware of bodily sensations or changes
      (b) Sometimes I am aware of bodily sensations or changes
      (c) I am often aware of bodily sensations or changes
      (d) I am constantly aware of bodily sensations or changes

4.   (a) Resisting thoughts of illness is never a problem
      (b) Most of the time I can resist thoughts of illness
      (c) I try to resist thoughts of illness but am often unable to do so
      (d) Thoughts of illness are so strong that I no longer even try to resist them

5.   (a) As a rule I am not afraid that I have a serious illness
      (b) I am sometimes afraid that I have a serious illness
      (c) I am often afraid that I have a serious illness
      (d) I am always afraid that I have a serious illness

6.   (a) I do not have images (mental pictures) of myself being ill
      (b) I occasionally have images of myself being ill
      (c) I frequently have images of myself being ill
      (d) I constantly have images of myself being ill

7. (a) I do not have any difficulty taking my mind off thoughts about my health
   (b) I sometimes have difficulty taking my mind off thoughts about my health
   (c) I often have difficulty in taking my mind off thoughts about my health
   (d) Nothing can take my mind off thoughts about my health

8. (a) I am lastingly relieved if my doctor tells me there is nothing wrong
   (b) I am initially relieved but the worries sometimes return later
   (c) I am initially relieved but the worries always return later
   (d) I am not relieved if my doctor tells me there is nothing wrong

9. (a) If I hear about an illness I never think I have it myself
   (b) If I hear about an illness I sometimes think I have it myself
   (c) If I hear about an illness I often think I have it myself
   (d) If I hear about an illness I always think I have it myself

10. (a) If I have a bodily sensation or change I rarely wonder what it means
    (b) If I have a bodily sensation or change I often wonder what it means
    (c) If I have a bodily sensation or change I always wonder what it means
    (d) If I have a bodily sensation or change I must know what it means

11. (a) I usually feel at very low risk for developing a serious illness
    (b) I usually feel at fairly low risk for developing a serious illness
    (c) I usually feel at moderate risk for developing a serious illness
    (d) I usually feel at high risk for developing a serious illness

12. (a) I never think I have a serious illness
    (b) I sometimes think I have a serious illness
    (c) I often think I have a serious illness
    (d) I usually think that I am seriously ill

13. (a) If I notice an unexplained bodily sensation I don't find it difficult to think about other things
    (b) If I notice an unexplained bodily sensation I sometimes find it difficult to think about other things
    (c) If I notice an unexplained bodily sensation I often find it difficult to think about other things
    (d) If I notice an unexplained bodily sensation I always find it difficult to think about other things

14. (a) My family/friends would say I do not worry enough about my health
    (b) My family/friends would say I have a normal attitude towards my health
    (c) My family/friends would say I worry too much about my health
    (d) My family/friends would say I am a hypochondriac

For the following questions, please think about what it would be like if you had a serious illness of a type which particularly concerns you (such as heart disease, cancer, multiple sclerosis, and so on). Obviously, you cannot know for definite what it would be like; please give your best estimate of what you *think* might happen, basing your estimate on what you know about yourself and serious illness in general.

---

15. (a) If I had a serious illness I would still be able to enjoy things in my life quite a lot
    (b) If I had a serious illness I would still be able to enjoy things in my life a little
    (c) If I had a serious illness I would be almost completely unable to enjoy things in my life
    (d) If I had a serious illness I would be completely unable to enjoy my life at all

16. (a) If I developed a serious illness there is a good chance that modern medicine would be able to cure me
    (b) If I developed a serious illness there is a moderate chance that modern medicine would be able to cure me
    (c) If I developed a serious illness there is a very small chance that modern medicine would be able to cure me
    (d) If I developed a serious illness there is no chance that modern medicine would be able to cure me

17. (a) A serious illness would ruin some aspects of my life
    (b) A serious illness would ruin many aspects of my life
    (c) A serious illness would ruin almost every aspect of my life
    (d) A serious illness would ruin every aspect of my life

18. (a) If I had a serious illness I would not feel that I had lost my dignity
    (b) If I had a serious illness I would feel that I had lost a little of my dignity
    (c) If I had a serious illness I would feel that I had lost quite a lot of my dignity
    (d) If I had a serious illness I would feel that I had totally lost my dignity

---

Each item on the questionnaire is scored on a scale from 0–3 (i.e., a = 0, b = 1, c = 2, d = 3). Add up the numbers to get your total score. In the original study from when this questionnaire was developed, patients with illness anxiety had an average total score of around 30 on this questionnaire; patients with other anxiety disorders (i.e., not illness anxiety) scored around 15, and individuals without anxiety scored around 9. What did you score? Were you closer to individuals with illness anxiety or individuals without?

If you are scoring high on this measure, you are not alone! Most of the estimates of the prevalence of illness anxiety/hypochondriasis diagnoses come from surveys of patients presenting to primary care clinics. Among patients in primary care, around 2–3% of people have diagnosable illness anxiety.[38, 39] In addition, up to 13% of people have recurrent anxiety about health that they find distressing.[39] If you take a moment to think about it, that's extremely common. That would mean that in any crowd of people, there are certain to be others who also have excessive worry about their health.

Motivation: Why Should I Take the Risk?

Working on changing anxious behaviors and thoughts is not easy. It is not just reading this book. It requires the willingness to try new behaviors and accept some level of risk in doing so. Along with that, it also requires a lot of time and effort spent in self-reflecting and completing the elements of this workbook, which involves actively changing your behavior and doing challenging tasks. It is important to weigh out the pros and cons of changing to see whether now is the right time for you to work on reducing illness anxiety.

Now, you may say to yourself, "I hate this anxiety, and I want it to go away! Of course I am motivated!" However, we think that *motivation* to change is not the same thing as *desire* to change. Most people reading this book will have the desire to change: that is, they recognize that their illness-related anxiety is causing them discomfort and they want to alleviate it. However, that is a very different thing from motivation to change, which to us is a willingness to tolerate some distress in the pursuit of your values. What does this mean? Change does not happen easily—at a minimum, it requires regular devotion of time for practice, and can be emotionally difficult at times. To benefit from this program, you will have to *work* the program: take your time to carefully self-reflect and complete the worksheets and exercises even if you think they are missing the mark, and be mindful of your daily actions to take opportunities to practice change. In addition, doing treatment when you are not ready or when it does not work for you may lead you to avoid treatment in the future or feel that treatment cannot help you or make you less likely to stick with it in the future,[40] even though it may certainly help when the time is right! Therefore, considering whether the cost is worth the benefit for you right now is crucial. You may decide that now is not the best time to work on your illness anxiety—and that's OK. Return to the program when you feel like you have the resources and willingness to devote to it.

To begin to consider whether this program is worth it for you right now, we encourage you to take an honest inventory of the pros and cons of working on changing your behavior at this time. We encourage this simple exercise even if you feel that you are ready and willing to change. Taking a thorough motivation inventory at the beginning can help so you have on hand when your motivation falters in the future (as it does for nearly everyone at times). This inventory often starts with a reflection on what you think the anxiety problem has taken from you, or what consequences it has led to in your life. This is often very different for different people. Also, often people have gotten so used to living with anxiety that they don't realize that things may be improved. Or people may be minimizing the impact of their anxiety on themselves and others because it is difficult to face.

What Problems Has My Anxiety Caused Me?
First, take a moment to consider what problems health anxiety has contributed to for you, and what problems may arise or

continue if you decide to not work on it at this time. Below, we included a list of some of the most common things that people have told us they hate about their excessive anxiety about health. We encourage you to read the list carefully and elaborate on the consequences you think may apply to you, as well as the level of distress and impact it has had on your life.

The most immediate consequences that come to mind first for most people are the psychological consequences: the distress and discomfort that anxiety can create.

Psychological Distress

How often do you feel distressed by your health-related anxiety? If you had to put it all together, how much of your average day in (in minutes or hours) is taken up by the anxiety or health-related thoughts?

_____

_____

Often people report frustration with their anxious thoughts, stating that they feel that they cannot enjoy activities as much as they used to, and feel less able to be spontaneous and tolerate new activities. Sometimes they give up activities that they previously enjoyed, such as yoga, walking, seeing friends, or biking, as they fear worsening or triggering medical symptoms or worries. Since your worries started, have you given up on any activities that you previously used to do?

_____

_____

People may also start to lose a sense of self-confidence that they can tolerate difficult or anxiety-inducing situations. They might report that their world keeps getting smaller as they work to avoid anxiety.

Do you think this sounds like you? How so? In what other ways does the illness anxiety impact your mental well-being?

_____

_____

_____

_____

_____

Interpersonal Impact

Anxiety also often leads to interpersonal consequences, such as others becoming frustrated with our expressions of anxiety or relentless requests for reassurance.

How do your family members react to your anxiety? Do they accommodate you by providing you with excessive reassurance or helping you avoid situations that bother you? Are they understanding and supportive? Do they criticize, or become frustrated?

_____

_____

_____

_____

How do your close friends and acquaintances act? Do they know about your anxiety?

_____

_____

_____

_____

Because it can be difficult to identify the impact your anxiety has had on others, if you are comfortable asking those who know you well, we encourage you to survey close friends or relatives. You can ask them about what anxious behaviors they have seen in you, and how your health anxiety may impact them. If you are comfortable with this exercise, we have included a template below of questions you may want to ask them. You can give them the form to complete, or you can simply ask them the questions. Obviously, do not survey your friends/loved ones if you think doing so will lead to adverse consequences (e.g., arguments, discomfort with having shared your anxiety). If you survey others, you must be ready and open to receiving their direct, honest feedback.

Person 1 (their relationship to you): _____

Please honestly complete the questions below about your loved one or friend. Please remember to be kind in order to provide constructive feedback and not shame your loved one.

Have you noticed how your (friend/family/partner)'s anxiety about health has changed them? If yes, please describe: What have you seen that tells you they are anxious about health? Do you see any behaviors that concern you?

_____

_____

_____

_____

_____

How does your (friend/family/partner)'s health anxiety impact your life? Do you do anything differently because they are anxious, such as provide them with reassurance, avoid talking about certain topics, help them with anxious behaviors, allow them to avoid certain tasks, or any other things you would not do if they did not have anxiety?

_____

_____

_____

_____

_____

Person 2 (their relationship to you): _____

Please honestly complete the questions below about your loved one or friend. Please remember to be kind in order to provide constructive feedback and not shame your loved one.

Have you noticed how your (friend/family/partner)'s anxiety about health has changed them? If yes, please describe: What have you seen that tells you they are anxious about health? Do you see any behaviors that concern you?

_____

_____

_____

_____

_____

How does your (friend/family/partner)'s health anxiety impact your life? Do you do anything differently because they are anxious, such as provide them with reassurance, avoid talking about certain topics, help them with anxious behaviors, allow them to avoid certain tasks, or any other things you would not do if they did not have anxiety?

_____

_____

_____

_____

_____

Behavioral Efforts

On average, how much time do you spend in a day in health-related activities (or avoiding health-related activities!), such as monitoring your health in various ways, researching, or asking about health, doctor's visits, actively attempting to distract yourself from health anxiety, or talking about health, etc.? What exactly do you do?

_____

_____

_____

Financial Costs

Having illness anxiety can be expensive, in time and money. Individuals with health anxiety are more likely than those without it to seek and receive costly healthcare services. They visit primary care doctors more,[41] obtain more medical tests, see more specialists,[42] and go to the emergency room or urgent care more often.[43, 44] Occasionally, people have spent lots of money on unnecessary doctors' visits, alternative or adjunctive treatments, second opinions, extra medical tests, medications they have not used, vitamins, and more.

Have there been any financial costs to you as a result of your anxiety about health? How much do you think you have spent in total, or on a regular basis? If you did not have to spend your money on your health, what would you prefer to spend it on instead?

_____

_____

_____

Work-related Impact

Illness anxiety is associated with more days of not attending work, difficulty completing work-related responsibilities, and more frequent reliance on disability benefits.[45, 46] Do you think your anxiety has impacted your work performance at all? Have you ever had to miss work because of it (i.e., because you were too anxious, or needed to attend a medical appointment)? If yes, please describe below:

_____

_____

_____

Medical Backfiring

Have you had to avoid treatments that your doctors recommended to you, because of your anxiety about the treatment or side effects? What were you concerned would happen? Have there been negative consequences for avoiding the medical treatments that were recommended?

_____

_____

_____

_____

Have you requested additional testing that may lead to higher likelihood of benign issues being discovered? Or have your requested additional testing or procedures that may even be harmful (e.g., extra x-rays or antibiotics)?

_____

_____

_____

How do you think your doctor perceives you—do they possibly think you are anxious and difficult to deal with? Do you think this impacts how they treat you? For example, do you think they are less likely to listen to you or more likely to dismiss your symptoms as anxiety? Or are they more likely to give you unnecessary testing and procedures to try and appease you?

Increasing Awareness with Self-monitoring

The first step of any good CBT is to increase awareness. You may already think that you have a good understanding of your anxiety. For example, you might think, "I have suffered with this for a long time, and I worry about it every day; I know what I am anxious about!" However, we still need to gather more detail. We encourage you to do this by self-monitoring your episodes of anxiety, keeping a written log of anxious situations and responses.

There are many good reasons for doing this. First, it has the benefit of increasing personal awareness. We may be overestimating how well we know what triggers our anxiety and how good our recall is on our specific behavioral responses. Many thoughts and behaviors become so habitual that we may not even be aware of these processes as they occur. A monitoring log can begin to help us be more aware of subtle patterns in triggers, ways of thinking, or behaviors that can become specific targets for treatment. If you are in treatment with a therapist for illness anxiety, this record can also be extremely helpful in aiding your provider in formulating a treatment plan and tailoring treatment to your specific flavor of anxiety. In addition, it can help us track progress over time as we see how the monitoring may change as you progress through treatment. Finally, many patients of ours have said that the logs are a helpful record to have after treatment, in that they can review their responses. In doing so, they often realize how exaggerated their worries seemed. Reviewing the log regularly can help them keep in mind that at times of strong worry the anxiety seemed very realistic, but later in a cooler moment these thoughts are seen as irrational and extreme.

The best way to complete the self-monitoring is to take the monitoring form with you and fill it out when you notice that you are feeling distress related to your health worries. It is best if the monitoring is done in real time. We recognize that it is not always possible to do in the moment: for example, you may be driving, or in an important business meeting, and it may not be feasible to break out the form and hold up the conversation to begin to jot down your worries! However, we encourage you to write them down as soon as possible after the episode of distress. The reason for doing the monitoring in real time is that the more time between the event and the logging, the more thoughts tend to become distorted, and the less accurately we tend to remember the situation. Therefore, an important part of monitoring is to get more accurate data in the moment, or as soon as possible afterwards. Therefore, many people will carry the monitoring template with them to record their thoughts throughout the day. Some people will record the monitoring information in their phone or something else they always have with them, and then transfer the information to the log at the end of the day. However, if you are doing this, make sure that you get all the information needed, in sufficient detail. It is tempting to make a brief note in your phone—e.g., "anxious about my cold"—and not provide all the nuanced detail that is needed, like the specific content of the thought. It's important to know the words that you were telling yourself in your head, as if you were thinking out loud—for example, "I am having difficulty breathing. The doctor said this was a cold but what if they are wrong? I should go back to Urgent Care just to be sure. I can't sit with this discomfort or I will go crazy."

Below is the template that we typically use for monitoring, with a couple of example entries already completed to give you a sense of what it might look like. In column one, you will identify the situation that started the anxiety. Almost always, if we pay close attention, there is some kind of trigger for our anxiety/worry, even if it was an intrusive thought or subtle signal. Part of using the self-monitoring log is to get a better sense of what some of these trigger patterns might be. However, sometimes it seems like the anxiety seemed to pop out of the blue. If you can't identify a specific event that got the anxiety going, just try to note what was going on at the time—for example, who you were with, where you were, and what you were doing right before you noticed the anxiety kick up.

In the second column, you will write down the thoughts that you had in response to the trigger. In this column, try to write down literally what you are saying to yourself in your head. Therefore, rather than just writing down something vague such as, "I noticed a pain and was anxious it might be something serious," write down the specific thought, such as, "I noticed that I was having pains in my left arm, and my doctor recently told me that this might be a sign of heart disease in women. I may be having a heart attack right now."

Once you write down the thoughts that you are having, then try to dig down another layer by asking yourself, if that scary outcome were true, what would be the scariest part about that feared outcome to you? For example, what would be so bad if an arm pain was a heart attack? Not everyone would agree on what is the scariest part about such an outcome. Some people might say, "I will drop dead suddenly and leave my family uncared for." Some people might say, "I will not know where to go or what do to for help," and so on.

Take a moment now to make a practice entry or two with a recent episode of health anxiety that you had.

Health Anxiety Monitoring Form

Trigger (What started the anxiety? Or what was going on at the time that you noticed your anxiety spike?)	Thoughts (Then, if that were true, what would be so bad about that?)	Distress level (0–10)
I woke up after another night of poor sleep after several nights in a row.	I remember reading somewhere that lack of sleep is related to lowered immune function for people my age. This is going to make it more likely I get severely ill and end up in the hospital, where I will be likely to catch even more illnesses.	6

Trigger (What started the anxiety? Or what was going on at the time that you noticed your anxiety spike?)	Thoughts (Then, if that were true, what would be so bad about that?)	Distress level (0–10)
I noticed a small rash-like mark on my neck.	I haven't seen anything like this before. I should call the doctor. It might be something serious and if I don't catch it early, it could become something untreatable and fatal.	5

Take a look at your practice entry. Did you write your thoughts out in as much detail as possible, writing what your interpretation of the scary scenario was, and adding why it would be truly awful to you if this outcome was true or occurred?

Make sure to "listen" to your thoughts and write down what you are telling/implying to yourself in your head—how you talk to yourself about these things is important, as we will discuss in the next chapter. Then begin to record throughout the week.

If you find that you have many episodes of distress, you do not need to write out all of them if you feel like you will constantly be writing! Writing down a few significant episodes of distress will suffice to be able to detect some patterns. In addition, it is if you find yourself writing down the same types of things. We have found that sometimes patients will come back with only a couple entries in their monitoring log. We then express surprise, since it seems like they only felt anxious a couple times over the past week! They may then clarify that they felt anxious many times each day, but did not write down each instance because they were worried about the same types of things. In these cases, we encourage you to continue to write down significant episodes of distress even if you are writing similar things. Part of the monitoring is being able to identify patterns.

We recommend keeping the log for at least two weeks, to get a very good sense of what your anxiety patterns are, since your tailored treatment plan will rely on some of this information.

2

What Are My Problematic Health-related Beliefs?

What Are Your Illness Fears?

Have you been completing your self-monitoring log regularly? What are some patterns in the triggers and thoughts that you have listed? What is your brain telling you so you can feel more anxious?

Remember, anxiety likes to exist at all costs in our brain, it desperately wants to survive. An analogy we sometimes use in our clinical work is that of Ursula in *The Little Mermaid* (the older cartoon). She has these small shrimps she eats, and they continue to make her large and physically strong. One could imagine Ursula as your anxiety and your anxious thoughts as the shrimps. Every time she eats, she gets stronger. Thus, every time you have an anxious thought, your anxiety gets stronger. So the goal is to starve your anxiety bully (Ursula) to make her as weak as possible in order to defeat her. By not feeding anxiety with anxious thoughts, we can weaken its power.

As we have already mentioned, it's important to first get a sense of what about the illness process is especially frightening for you. It may seem like it should be obvious, as the general ideas of death, dying, and illness are scary for almost everybody! However, different people make different sense of what

DOI: 10.4324/9781032711355-2

the process of illness and/or dying may be like, and what may be especially catastrophic about it to them. For example, some people may be afraid of getting a chronic illness that would inhibit their physical movement and lead to prolonged disability and loss of aspects of independence. Some people are afraid of the idea of uncertainty, or images of nothingness that may come with thoughts of the afterlife. Some people are worried they will die suddenly, and that their loved ones will be left to care for themselves. These are just some examples. There are many different things that a person could be afraid of about the illness process. Usually there are one or two things that people might be especially afraid of, and these come in the form of our thoughts—or how we appraise a situation, feeling, environment, or person.

Many people say, "I'm just afraid of dying!" However, in most cases, it's generally not as simple as being afraid of dying. People with illness anxiety often can recognize that they are not as afraid of dying in other ways, such as by sudden accident or other catastrophe; at least it doesn't haunt them on a daily basis the way that illness fears do. The absence of excessive fears about other forms of dying is a sign that the fear is not of the process of dying itself, but rather some aspect of illness that bothers you. Usually, it is a theme associated with fear of disability, uncontrollability of random illness, and so on. It's also not just a fear of "getting ill"—individuals with illness anxiety also often state that they are generally not afraid of illnesses if there are some mitigating factors; some examples may be if they know the diagnosis or at least have a plan of treatment, they know the disease is not fatal, or they know it will end. In that case, one may be afraid of tolerating uncertainty.

Tolerating uncertainty is a difficult concept to grasp, and when we first bring it up related to health, many people are resistant to doing so. However, if you were to look at your week and see how much of it was uncertain (or unpredictable), you would see that you actually have very little control and you already tolerate a high level of uncertainty in your life—we just don't think we do! It can be a very motivating task to work through the chart below and realize you already have a skill you just need to apply to your illness anxiety.

Using the Downward Arrow to Further Identify
Your Anxious Appraisals and Thoughts

Although it can seem like you think about your feared out-comes all the time, we don't typically think through the scariest aspects of our fears in tons of detail. Therefore, we may not be entirely aware of what about the idea of illness is so scary for us. Sometimes we think that trying to avoid anxious thoughts is the best thing to avoid our anxiety, but in fact, it's the opposite. By not facing your anxious thoughts, you are reinforcing to your brain that they are something scary and you need to fear them. In reality, anxious thoughts are just scary, nasty thoughts that don't have to mean anything or be acted on.

We can use a technique called the downward arrow to probe what some of the scary predictions may be for you. It's OK as you go through this if you are unsure of the answers to the questions, but we encourage you to try your best to really think through the situation and speculate. Most people, once they get to a certain point in the down arrow, have trouble answering the questions, as people rarely think through their anxious fears in this much detail. We highly encourage you to go through this process even if you think you already know what your feared outcome is, as the treatment later will use some of these elements.

The downward arrow starts with a situation you fear and asks, "What would be so bad about that?" It's best to start with a situation that makes you so anxious that you avoid it or use lots of protective behaviors to help yourself feel better about it. Then you will ask yourself, "What would happen if I entered this situation without any protective behaviors? For example, what would happen if I went to the doctor without preparing before I went? What would happen if I stopped using my digital activity tracker? Stopped checking my pulse and blood pressure? Stopped asking others for health reassurance?"

Once you have identified what is so bad about not avoiding, the process is repeated, asking yourself, "Well, if even that were true, what would be so bad about *that*?" This continues for at least a few layers. Using this method can help people identify what some of their scary appraisals are of their feared situation.

This process can be difficult, so before you attempt yours, you can read through some of the examples below. It is also entirely normal if you feel some discomfort while thinking about and assessing your appraisals.

A tip for doing the downward arrow: try not to use emotions as feared outcomes (e.g., "I would feel anxious") unless the emotional experience itself is the *only* feared outcome you can identify. Rather, really try to ask yourself, "Why would I feel this emotion—what sense am I making of this situation, or what prediction am I making, that would lead me to feel this way?"

Sometimes the experience of emotions alone *is* the only feared outcome, however, even if we might not even be able to think of a reason why we would feel that emotion in the situation. Sometimes we are simply anxious about being anxious, fearful of the subjective experience of being disgusted, or so on. In that case, continue the downward arrow, asking yourself what about the emotional experience is so bad, as in the example below. Even with emotional experiences, we may fear them for different reasons and make different senses of them. Sometimes people are simply fearful of having strong emotions, and in this case it is usually because they are implying to themselves that something will happen if they do not try to check the emotions, such as having a breakdown, having an embarrassing loss of control, the emotion becoming permanent, or something similar.

Now try to complete your own downward arrow in Figure 2.3a. Again, it usually works best if you start with asking what would happen if you gave up a safety behavior (e.g., refrained from excessively checking health, or other behaviors to try to control health).

Take a look at your downward arrow: do you think most of your safety/avoidance behaviors relate to this feared outcome? If not, you may want to do another downward arrow using Figure 2.3b with the behavior that you think may have a different feared outcome:

Example 1:

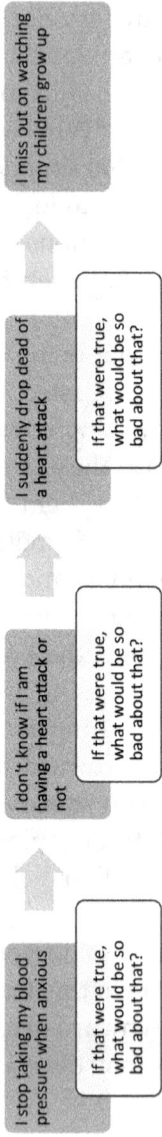

Example 2:

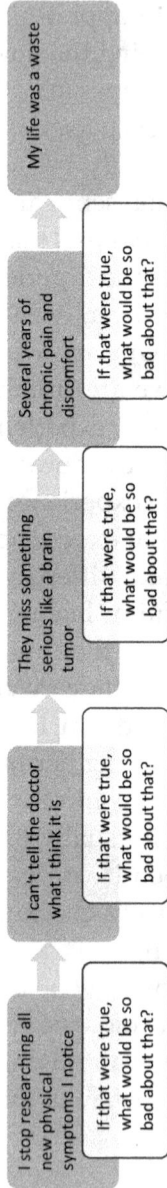

FIGURE 2.1 Downward arrow examples

Example 3:

I stop trying to figure out my symptoms

If that were true, what would be so bad about that?

I always feel uncertain as to whether my symptoms are serious or not

If that were true, what would be so bad about that?

Anxiety that never goes away or increases over time

If that were true, what would be so bad about that?

I never enjoy life again

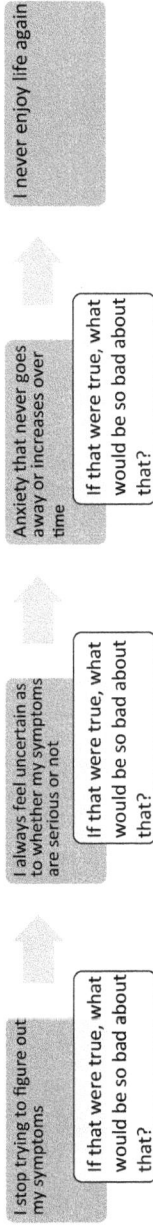

FIGURE 2.2 Downward arrow example 3

If that were true, what would be so bad about that?

If that were true, what would be so bad about that?

If that were true, what would be so bad about that?

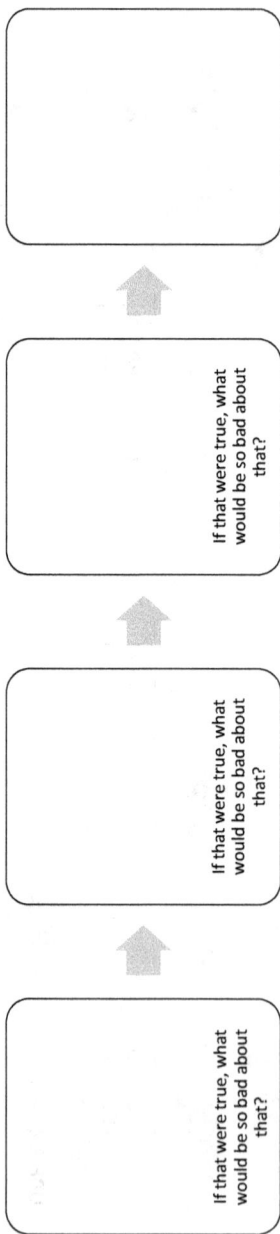

FIGURE 2.3A Blank downward arrow

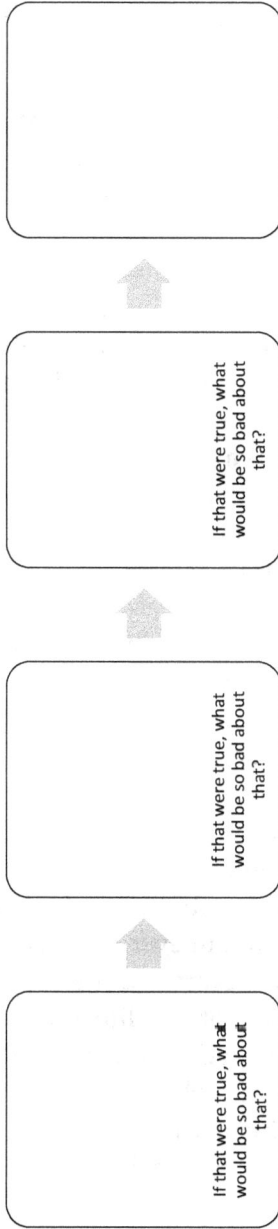

FIGURE 2.3B Blank downward arrow

Box 1: If that were true, what would be so bad about that?

Box 2: If that were true, what would be so bad about that?

Box 3: If that were true, what would be so bad about that?

When You Are Anxious, You Are Not Thinking Clearly

When we are anxious, the feeling that danger is imminent can be very overwhelming and loud. Danger feels very real and imminent. However, it is often just that—a feeling. It may not necessarily match with what we believe, or what is realistic given the evidence available to us. In fact, it is usually not completely accurate. If you think about it, while feelings are an important source of information (they are there to guide us, after all), they can be quite faulty. For example, a depressed person may feel worthless, but that does not necessarily mean that he or she has no worth. A person with contamination fears-based OCD may feel very afraid that if they do not wash their hands every ten minutes, they will get ill. We may *feel* that someone in a court case is guilty, even when there is a lack of concrete evidence, but there is a reason why we can't convict people for crimes that we simply feel they are guilty of! Just because emotions are strong does not mean that they are accurate.

We often feel emotions for reasons that are unexplainable or not obvious to us, for reasons such as conditioning. For those of you who may have missed Psych 101 class, conditioning occurs when things get paired together by association. This is what makes your dog or cat come running when they hear the can opener—they have learned that every time they hear the noise of a can opener, dinnertime shortly follows! Similar conditioning happens in humans quite often, and can happen outside our full awareness. For example, say that all through school I really hated math and struggled with it in every math class that came along. Also, perhaps by chance, every math teacher I had was a petite woman with blonde hair. Later in life, I may feel weird, anxious, or irritable around short, petite women with blonde hair, for reasons that are unclear to me! However, it was because of the random and repeated pairing of these two things, not because petite women who are blonde math teachers are inherently dangerous or awful!

This is one reason why we can have strong emotions that feel valid, but can often simultaneously recognize on an intellectual level that they do not make complete sense. As another example, imagine an untouched clear glass of water, and next to it, another glass of water with a cockroach in it that had been completely sterilized. Even if it was possible to assure you that the bug in the water could not touch you in any way or contaminate the water in any way, almost everyone would have a strong feeling of disgust and choose to drink from the clear water! To go even further, most people would report having no desire to drink from the cockroach glass even after it had been cleaned in soap and water, despite cognitively knowing that there were no germs present. In cases like this, people can often recognize that the task (e.g., drinking from the bug glass) is not inherently dangerous. However, they are stopped by a strong feeling of disgust. We have these feelings based on conditioning (i.e., our brains making these associations) because it helped keep our ancestors alive. Also, we are taught these things, via modeling and learning. Generally speaking, it makes sense to be wary about consuming creepy crawlies, and this is a general "rule" that Western society follows and teaches: bugs are gross and should be avoided. Therefore this response is somewhat hardwired, and the "avoid" feeling is quite strong. However, that does not mean that all bugs are dangerous or germy, in all settings, and at all times. In fact, in some cultures bugs are part of the regular diet and are not at all viewed as dangerous or germy! Now, we are not saying that you need to drink bug water to overcome your illness anxiety(!), but rather we are using this example to encourage you to step back and evaluate your thoughts and behaviors to determine if they rationally make sense to you, or if they are a way of behaving that is overly based on emotion. Often our rules for safety become overgeneralized—that is, they become rigid and way more comprehensive than they need to be. As another example, consider someone who develops posttraumatic stress disorder after being sexually assaulted by a male in an elevator. Due to the intense fear of the association with the scary event and the situation, they may subsequently avoid all elevators and men, fearing that they are dangerous. While the assault was awful and some protective behaviors may be appropriate, the extent of avoidance is an example of not-so-adaptive overgeneralization based on strong feelings: feeling that because a bad event happened in this context, all men and elevators are to be avoided. The rule is designed to protect, but has become too broad to be useful, is hindering one from living a full life, and is maintaining a feeling that the world is dangerous.

Our brains have evolved to maintain this phenomenon in a couple of ways. First, our fight or flight system becomes highly active when we are feeling an intense emotion like anxiety. Simultaneously, our pre-frontal cortex (the logic, reason, and decision-making part of the brain) starts to function differently.[1-3] This means that when we are highly anxious, we are not relying as heavily on the rational part of our brain, so the impact is that we can know logically that something is not dangerous, but we can feel very frightened and act as if the thing is dangerous while feeling afraid. This is one reason why no amount of reassurance when you feel anxious feels quite good enough. Evolutionarily, this neurological process is quite helpful. For example, if we run into a bear in the woods, we don't want to stop and carefully think through all the pros and cons of our options. In the time that could take, you could very well get mauled by the bear. Instead, our body de-emphasizes that analytical part of our brain and reacts to keep us safe. Though adaptive, this can serve to maintain avoidance behaviors in illness anxiety.

Despite feelings making our fears seem very real, and despite our feeling confident in our conclusions, there are many ways that we are thinking when we are anxious that are biased. Often, we are not even aware that this is happening. Maybe you have heard the phrase "rose-colored glasses" to describe people who are overly optimistic. Being anxious is like wearing gray-colored glasses—it colors the world darkly, filtering things through a negative light. In the next section, we describe many ways in which thinking can become distorted related to health.

Catastrophizing: Overestimating the Likelihood and Severity of Feared Outcomes

No doubt, when you are anxious, the things you are afraid of seem like very real and scary things that can happen to you.

When people have excessive anxiety, they tend to overestimate the likelihood of scary things happening, and often think those situations or events will be much more severe and awful than they typically are.[4-7] It is not unusual for anxious individuals to worry about something for years and years, only to find that if their feared outcome happens, it is underwhelming compared with what they were anticipating. People often underestimate their ability to cope with negative things that could happen to them. But most often, people spend a lifetime worrying about things that never happen!

This overestimation of how likely bad things are, and how bad they will be if they were to occur, is called "catastrophizing." You may have heard this term before, as it's been used in CBT for many years. It's been shown to be a common thinking pattern that people have when they are anxious. This thinking style has also been shown to actively worsen anxiety problems. However, like many ways of thinking when we are anxious, it can be quite inaccurate and lead us down an unhelpful path. One common sign that you might be engaging in catastrophic thinking is if you are using the phrase, "What if …?" Usually in these instances we are trying to plan for the worst.

Catastrophizing is one of the most common thinking distortions that comes up when people are worried about health. Chances are you can remember a time when your health anxiety had taken over your brain: it likely felt that health disaster was imminent. During these times, people tend to overestimate how likely health outcomes actually are. These overestimations of feared outcomes are often specific to severe or fatal illnesses, while your estimations of routine and benign illnesses may be more accurate.

In addition to overestimating how probable health problems are, people also tend to overestimate how bad the situation will be, and overestimate (as compared with non-health-anxious people) how much responsibility they have for preventing feared health outcomes.[4] When anxious, we are generally assuming a worst-case scenario: painful death, fatal diagnoses we cannot cope with, emotional breakdowns, prolonged disability, and so on. Sometimes there is vivid imagery that goes along with this:

lying in a hospital bed alone with profound pain and hopeless-ness, having to give up all fun activities and no longer enjoying life, crying family members living a lifetime of grief. Extreme outcomes like this are always *possible*. We know that you likely are grimacing after reading that, but it is in your best interest to confront the fears rather than running from them. In life, we do have to coexist with the potential for very serious negative out-comes. However, we have found that in the rare cases when peo-ple do eventually experience a serious health crisis, they often find that they cope with the situation much better than antici-pated and the situation was not at all how they imagined it. As with most anxiety disorders, we can get stuck on the serious but extremely rare potential negative outcomes. This can easily lead to a life spent worrying about things that do not happen, or at least not how we imagined them.

Your Health-related Attentional Biases

When we are anxious, we tend to filter incoming information—what we see and hear—through a lens of paying attention to danger. We selectively pay attention to things that make us anx-ious, which leads to our noticing them more! Let's take an exam-ple that is not related to medical disease but that many of us can relate to: fear of spiders. Someone who has a strong phobia of spi-ders might report that they see them every week or even every day—much more than everyone else—because they are paying more attention to dark corners and checking holes where spiders might live. In a similar way, you pay more attention to things that are relevant to your health fears,[8] making it seem like health danger is everywhere. Because individuals with illness anxiety are so vigilant to health problems, they have often inadvertently trained themselves to be good noticers of symptoms. They have good interoceptive or internal awareness[9]—which means they are likely to notice bodily symptoms before anyone else does. To a person with illness anxiety, that may sound like a good thing—after all, if you can detect symptoms or signs, you can act earlier, right? However, what happens is that people tend to notice benign signs and symptoms—routine fluctuations in bodily sensations, and catastrophize about them, assuming they are signs of something serious. Therefore, good interoceptive awareness can be *too* good, in that it can be associated with higher depression and anxiety.[10]

The media play a significant role in how people interpret things as well. During virus outbreaks—such as during the COVID pandemic—media reports about health issues become much more widespread. To get people to tune in, these media stories try to heighten emotions by describing worst-case scenarios and using scary language.[11] Unfortunately, people with illness anxiety are more likely to interpret symptoms in that context, for example assuming that benign and routine symptoms may be related to COVID exposure.[12]

Some research[13] has suggested that anxious people also have more difficulty disengaging from cues that suggest danger—and that illness-anxious people pay more attention to health-related information in general.[14–16] What this all means is that people who are anxious often notice and pay more attention to more information, they tend to remember it more, and then their world starts to seem very dangerous and scary. However, this doesn't mean that it is. It means it was *perceived* that way. Have you ever heard a Republican and a Democrat talk about a political debate they both have just watched? They may have completely different accounts of the same event! They perceive it in a filtered way—it is being processed consistent with their beliefs. Do not forget that everything you are perceiving is going through a filter of anxiety in which you are excessively looking for danger and finding it. This can color your reality in substantial ways. This is one of the main reasons looking at evidence is important for making conclusions about what course of action you'd like to take when it comes to your health, but also one of the major reasons why finding information that goes against our anxious beliefs is so hard. We have spent a long time looking for evidence that supports our anxious beliefs, and the feelings are so strong, that we often don't question them. Therefore, doing so is very hard—just like considering the merits of an alternative political viewpoint, it can make us feel very uncomfortable and be hard to consider all the "pros."

Underestimating Your Ability to Cope

In addition to over-estimating the likelihood and severity of feared outcomes, we often *under*-estimate our own ability to cope with these situations. Sometimes what makes these health scenarios seem so terrifying is that we are worried about how we (or others, sometimes) will cope with them. It is likely you can cite examples of times when you feel that you did not cope well with a loss, health scare, severe episode of anxiety or depression, or similar. You may have had past episodes of anxiety or depression and feel especially worried that they will come back, that you will handle them badly, or that you will have a full-on nervous breakdown and not be able to function! In short, sometimes we are making many negative predictions about how much anxiety we will have, and how much it will impact our life. If you think you might be having these thoughts as well, try to identify the specific predictions you are making, and write those down as a feared outcome as well.

We call these overly negative predictions "catastrophic thoughts," as they are often implying that the worst will happen. The presence of these catastrophic thoughts that overestimate the likelihood and severity of feared outcomes may not be obvious to you, since it is unlikely that you are sitting around calculating the precise probabilities of your feared outcomes happening to you. Take a moment to turn back to your completed downward arrow in Figures 2.3a and 2.3b. For each step of your downward arrow, write down a probability estimate of how likely you think this outcome is.

Below is an example of this with the steps of the downward arrow from Figures 2.1 and 2.2 earlier in this chapter:

Feared outcome:	My estimated probability:	Evidence for or against this outcome:
1) If I stop researching new physical symptoms, I won't be able to tell the doctor what I think it is.	30%	"I know sometimes after research I have caught things and brought them to my doctor's attention. But I usually have a sense of what it is before all the research."
2) Because I am unable to tell the doctor what I think it is, they will miss something important.	30%	"Again, I have brought things to their attention in the past which it seems like they weren't considering. However, this seems to not happen often. They may also eventually figure it out."
3) I am diagnosed with something serious, like a brain tumor.	10%	"Brain tumors get missed sometimes; I've seen it in the news. But the chances of my having a brain tumor are minor."
4) I have to live with several years of pain and discomfort after diagnosis of tumor.	40%	"I might die quickly, might recover, or might suffer for a while; all of these are possibilities I have heard happen to people with cancer."
5) My life was a waste because I had a tumor.	0%	"I recognize this is not true. My life would not be a waste just because it ended in cancer."

Now, fill in your predictions and estimates in the following worksheet. For now, hold off on the last column, labeled "Evidence for or against this feared outcome." We will come back to that in a moment.

Evidence Weighing Form

Feared outcome:	Estimated probability:	Evidence for or against this feared outcome:

Now that you have entered in your fearful predictions and estimated probabilities, let's take a double look at your probability estimates. Chances are, because you are anxious, your first estimates of probability were likely based on strong feelings, and not adequately noticing or factoring in evidence such as what you have been told by knowledgeable people, or what you have seen or experienced. Also, chances are that you are discounting information that goes against your fears, such as times when your feared outcomes did not occur, or incidences in which problems did not arise. Remember that when you are anxious, you are more likely to remember information that supports your fears rather than information that goes against them. That does not mean that other evidence is not there. It does, however, mean that you are out of practice in looking for it!

Think about your probabilities. A 30% estimate of the doctor missing something would mean that three in ten times I go to the doctor, the doctor misses something critical. A 40% estimate that you will get very bad news when you visit the doctor would mean that four in ten times you have gone to the doctor in the past, you have received bad news. Think about whether those estimates sound accurate to you based on your experience and what you know. Does the doctor give you horrible news every two in five visits? Revise your probability estimates if you think they are off. If you have loved ones you trust (who don't have illness anxiety themselves!), you may want to ask them if they would agree with your probabilities.

The final step is to go back to the Evidence Weighing Form and spend some time really thinking and filling out the last column, which is the evidence you have for or against this feared outcome. What data do you have to support or negate this feared outcome? Remember that you are more likely to have information that is consistent with your fears, so spend some careful time trying to be a lawyer for the other side of the case—the side arguing against your fears. As you try this case against your thoughts, the data you present should not be a strong feeling, but rather evidence that is "presentable in court," such as scientific data, expert testimony (make sure you are citing reputable sources, such as scientific outlets or well-known organizations), and things you have directly experienced, witnessed, or have expertise in. It should not include data from faulty sources, such as one-off cases you have heard about, individual and biased accounts such as nonscientific blogs or listservs, or comments from other anxious individuals. Without doing excessive research, try to include numbers and frequencies as much as possible—for example, rather than saying, "I know this is unlikely," say why: "I know of only one person this has happened to, ever." Or rather than saying, "It is unlikely I have meningitis," say "[scientific organization's website] says only 1/100,000 people each year have meningitis, and I have none of the risk factors."

Because you are viewing life through those gray-colored lenses when it comes to health, we know this will not be easy. The following is an example of the Evidence Weighing Form with the evidence column completed to give you a sense of what this might look like. As you do this exercise, really take time to consider what evidence you are drawing your conclusions from, and whether these are valid sources of information that can be used as evidence, or if they are hearsay or biased perception. Based on the data available, revise your probability estimates if necessary. You may also want to have someone you trust help you inventory possible evidence that you are not thinking of.

Evidence Weighing Form: Example

Feared outcome:	Estimated probability:	Evidence for and against this feared outcome:
1) If I stop re-searching new physical symptoms, I won't be able to tell the doctor what I think it is.	30%	In the past there have been a couple times I have mentioned something to my doctor and they have looked into it further. So maybe 3 out of 40 times I have been to the doctor. Once I really had to advocate to get my doctor to do some additional allergy testing and found that I did indeed have an allergy. My doctors usually can diagnose and treat me without my opinion. Most people I know don't do much research before they go to the doctor. I have asked them.

Feared outcome:	Estimated probability:	Evidence for and against this feared outcome:
2) Because I am unable to tell the doctor what I think it is, they will miss something important.	30%	My allergy was only caught after I asked several times and presented some research to the doctor. However, I don't know if it would have been caught eventually. There have been many other times (at least once a year) when I have not been able to tell my doctor what I thought the issue was, and those did not end up in a serious issue being found later.
3) I will be diagnosed with something serious, like a brain tumor.	10%	I do not have any of the risk factors for cancer/brain tumors. I do not have any current symptoms that would suggest a brain tumor. Tumors are a rare condition: (less than 1% of people) based on the scientific journals I looked up with my therapist
4) I will have to live with several years of pain and discomfort after diagnosis of tumor.	40%	The scientific journals said 20–66% of people survive at least five years, but also that there are over 100 types of brain tumors that all have different severity levels and prognoses. Some of them are sudden and fatal, but some are highly treatable and relatively benign. I have had at least three family members with cancer, and two of them had pain at the end. However, they functioned pretty well for years until then. One of them had a tumor, and they had it treated and are in remission now. They did not report much discomfort other than the surgery.
5) My life was a waste because I had a tumor	0%	My life is not defined by how it ends. I have done many generous, good things for people and have had a positive impact. I have also had lots of great experiences.

Did you notice any catastrophizing in your initial thinking patterns? If yes, that's typical! The first step is just to be aware that they are present and influencing how anxious you feel.

You may also notice that your estimated probabilities look different in the moment when anxiety is at its peak compared to when you have calmed down (maybe even on a different day). This is because our emotions color our estimates of probability.

Something we hear all too often is: "… but in the past when I didn't follow what my anxiety wanted me to do, there was something *actually* wrong. I can't trust myself." There is some truth to this statement. When anxiety starts to dictate our health decisions, we bias (focus) our attention to the specific signs or symptoms that confirm our fears. For example, if you are worried you have skin cancer, you are more likely to visually inspect your body, and therefore more likely to find skin blemishes or irregularities that you temporarily believe are cancerous. At the same time, because of thinking biases you will likely be dismissing or downplaying the times when you went to the dermatologist and upon examination they found nothing to be clinically concerning. You may still think you need to continue with your visual checks because something can change and it might be the one time you did not that led to a cancerous mole not being detected. You aren't wrong, but you aren't right either.

Optional Exercise: Calculating the Estimated Probability of Your Scariest Scenario

Once you feel fairly confident in your probability estimates, if you like you can calculate the likelihood of your worst-case scenario by multiplying the probability of the steps. To do this, break out a calculator and multiply the percentages by moving the decimal point two places to the left. When you get your answer, move the decimal point two places back to the right to get a percentage likelihood.

This is complicated math for many people, so Figure 2.4 shows an example. So if we use the example problem from the form on page 53 and 56, after estimating probabilities we might end up

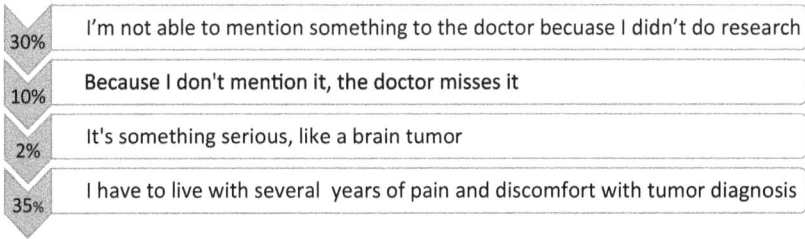

FIGURE 2.4 Probability downward arrow

estimating the probabilities shown in Figure 2.4 for the chain of feared events.

So to calculate the probability of the worst-case scenario occurring (the last step in the chain), you would move the decimal point two places to the left for each percentage estimate, and then multiply all of the probabilities together: .3 × .1 × .02 × .35. The answer is .00021. Move the decimal point back two places to the right for your final estimate: .021. What this means is that it is .021% likely that based on my probability estimates, I end up having to live with several years of pain and discomfort because of a tumor diagnosis that was undetected by a doctor because I failed to research and mention my findings to the doctor. This would be a 21 in 1,000 chance.

Keep in mind that because you are anxious, your estimates are still likely too high, but what do you think about this probability? You may say that the probability is so low that it is not worth the mental time and effort that you put into it. On some occasions, people do decide that the probability does seem relatively high, and there might be a real risk that needs a reasonable amount of practical attention. Sometimes appropriate preventative behaviors may be appropriate in rare cases if medical risk is high. What are your thoughts?

Sometimes these percentages and probabilities are hard to visualize. Below are some actual lifetime probability estimates from United States national data, for comparison.:

Negative health outcomes	Likelihood of this occurring in one's lifetime
Having a stroke under age 60	10% (1 in 10)[17]
Death from a car accident	1% (1 in 101)[18]
Pedestrian incident	.21% (1 in 485)[18]
Death from drowning	.10% (1 in 1,024)[18]
Death from choking	.03% (1 in 2,745)[18]
Death from a firearms accident	.012% (1 in 7,944)[18]
Being struck by lightening	.006% (1 in 15,300)[19]
Being bitten by a venomous snake	.002% (1 in 44,122)[20]
Death from anaphylaxis (serious allergic reaction)	.0006% (1 in 1,666,666)[21]
Death from a shark bite	.0004% (1 in 4 million)[21]

Let's take a closer look at these outcomes. Let's make sure you understand how these probabilities work (since probabilities in math is an area that most people have a hard time wrapping their heads around. There is a 1% chance you will die in a car accident, but does it mean that of the 100 times you have been in a car, that at least one of those times should have resulted in a car accident in which someone died? No—it means that roughly 1 in 100 people, on average, die in a car accident. Statistics, whether high or low, are just statistics. Unless the chances are 100%, your outcome is not set in stone. Also, since we love walking towards uncertainty rather than away from it, keep in mind that there are many factors that make these numbers go up or down, such as genetics, age, and lifestyle choices.

As anxiety tends to be irrational at times because of the biases we described above, often we are worrying about and protecting ourselves from things that are unlikely. We can practice talking back to these feelings, and acting according to what the facts are, while factoring in our emotions, but not necessarily letting them run the show. Are there any other things with similar outcomes to the ones that you are afraid of, such as disability, death, or unpredictability, that you do not protect yourself against as much as your specific health fears, despite it having a similar or even higher likelihood? What does this tell you?

3

What Are My Problematic Health-related Behaviors?

If you have been health-anxious for a while, you are likely behaving in ways that are different from other people when it comes to health. You likely fall into one of two categories: either *excessively avoiding* health-related information, or *excessively seeking* out reassurance and information about health conditions. Both response patterns in fact tend to maintain health-related anxiety over time. We will discuss methods for learning to approach health-related content for those who have a history of excessive avoidance, and we will discuss learning to adaptively reduce involvement in cases of excessive seeking of health-related content.

Before we teach methods for changing behavior, it is helpful to understand why these behaviors develop and stick around over time. Taken together, excessive approach and avoidance of health information are typically attempts to gain control over anxiety. For example, excessive information-seeking can result in a temporary, reinforcing feeling of reassurance that the doctor has not found anything, and excessive avoidance maintains the illusion that bad things will not happen if one doesn't know about them. Logically, we often know that our anxious behaviors and/or avoidance do not keep bad things from happening, but they provide a semblance of control and temporary relief. However, both excessive avoidance and excessive seeking may

DOI: 10.4324/9781032711355-3

have serious psychological consequences. Below we list some of the most common ones.

Potential Consequences of Excessive Health Information Seeking/avoidance:

♦ *It can be time-consuming!* It takes time to schedule appointments, find and maintain multiple providers, travel to appointments, check insurance coverage, participate in lab or other tests, or to research symptoms and results. This takes away from time doing other valued activities (work, hobbies, time with loved ones, etc.)

♦ *Increased sense of pessimism about health.* Excessive health seeking reinforces the fear that there is something wrong with our bodies and increases mistrust of our own ability to trust our bodies to keep us alive.

♦ *Mistrust of providers.* Both excessive avoidance and approach serve to decrease trust in providers. Avoidance reinforces the fear that providers are only going to share bad news, as people don't often test out what will happen if they consult with their providers more regularly and appropriately. Excessive approach, especially with multiple providers and Internet research, makes it difficult to trust that providers are accurately sharing information and have the proper expertise to treat whatever symptoms arise. It feeds into people's sense that they should be their own doctor, and leads to a lack of practice in trusting others.

♦ *Mistrust of your own judgment.* You likely viewed your symptoms and health experiences in a more realistic and manageable way prior to your health anxiety, if you can recall such a time. Now, noticing how you are often wrong when you make anxious predictions, you may feel unsure of when to be concerned about symptoms and when to wait it out. Some people report increased difficulties making decisions about health, along with reduced confidence in their judgments. This can be a frustrating experience.

◆ *Reduced confidence in our own ability to cope.* Anxiety makes it feel like bad outcomes are more likely than they are, and tries to convince us that we cannot handle it if bad things happen. With excessive avoidance or approach behaviors, we never get a chance to learn that we can handle so much more than we think we can. Rather, we continue to rely on distressing, consuming behaviors, thinking they are necessary for keeping us safe. It also prevents us from learning new coping skills for tolerating the unknown, anxiety, or bad news.

◆ *Increased focus on health symptoms.* The more attention we give something, the more magnified it feels in our scope of attention. Most people have had the experience of saying or writing a word over and over, or focusing on a word too hard on writing it and it starts to look really weird after a while, or no longer seem like a word. Similar distortions can happen with over-focus on our body. The more we focus on determining if something strange is occurring, the more attention we are going to pay to random sensations, and the bigger they are going to feel. In this way, people with illness anxiety tend to train themselves to be very good noticers of bodily disruption—ordinary and generally benign fluctuations in signs and symptoms. While we may have the same bodily disturbances, if you have health anxiety, you are more likely you notice them before I do, as you have likely trained yourself to do so, even if you weren't aware of it. However, this means that you are more likely to notice a symptom and think it's a sign of something serious. The famous example of this in psychology is the oft-cited "white bear" study,[1] in which the researchers told a group of participants to do their best to avoid thinking of a white bear, and told another group to think about a white bear intentionally. This study found that the group of people who were instructed to *avoid* thinking about the bear became obsessive about white bears, while the other group did not! The takeaway message is that the more you try to not think about something, the more you will notice thoughts about it. Therefore, attempting to not think about or pay attention to health anxiety also runs the risk of increasing focus on symptoms.

◆ *Negative interactions with your social support system.* While you may find you that asking others around you to change their behavior does not negatively impact your health, it can impact the quality of your social relationships. Others may become frustrated with requests to behave according to your anxious rule book, or annoyed with repeat requests for health-related reassurance. Sometimes social relationships become overly focused on discussions of health issues, such that people become out of practice in how to talk about other things in life!

I recently had a [health-anxious] patient who decided that they never respond well to medications, and had side effects, so they changed to a Chinese herbal medicine for about three weeks, and sure enough they went into heart failure. It shocks me because they come and they just don't understand that it's because they are not taking the medication that's prescribed.

Dr L., Internal Medicine

There are parents [of child patients] that are totally unaware of how excessive they are: they ask all these questions, and I tell them [the child is] fine, but they won't take my word for it. They've googled something: 'it could be this, or it could be this.' I name off: 'her exam is normal, her oxygen is normal, you can come back if things get worse,' and might try to get up from my seat and move towards the door. There are more rarely people who request different tests that are outside what normal practice is, and you can get some pushback: 'I read about this test and I want to get it done.' I reiterate that based on my exam, vital signs, and your history, it would be extremely rare to have anything more serious, but they don't take my word for it.

Dr. L., Pediatrician

Identifying health-related behaviors that you may be excessively engaging in can be difficult. Sometimes people do not realize that they are engaging in these behaviors, or do not see that some of these behaviors may be classified as ways of avoiding. Sometimes avoidance can be subtle, but it is important to start to become aware of the ways (overt or subtle) that avoidance may be occurring. Below is a long list of health-related behaviors we have seen people do to try and get a sense of control over their health when they are feeling anxious. Many of them are appropriate in moderation, although most are not *necessary* to keep yourself healthy. However, these are behaviors that usually become excessive over time when we are anxious, and that perpetuate feelings of anxiety, even if they might feel helpful or otherwise relieving in the short term. We encourage you to go through the list, honestly self-reflect, and check off any behaviors you think you may engage in. We will come back to these later when talking about how to formulate a plan to work on these behaviors.

Health Behaviors Checklist

Reassurance Seeking
☐ Asking others about whether you should be worried about a particular physical symptoms or what treatment you should seek
☐ Talking about your health excessively
☐ Bringing up health issues to see if others are alarmed or not (includes just looking at the person's facial expressions in response to health news)
☐ Asking health questions even when you are pretty sure you know what the other person is going to say
☐ Excessively clicking on/reading Internet links/ads about illness, medical treatments, or people who had castastrophic medical issues
☐ Reading medical journal articles geared towards providers or scientists in the field

Doctor Seeking

☐ Making doctor appointments or seeking specialists that were not directly recommended by a doctor you are seeing

☐ Seeing several doctors and not adequately allowing them to share records/communicate

☐ Seeing too many doctors (e.g., seeing more than one doctor for an issue at once, or having too many doctors involved)

☐ Seeking second (or third!) medical opinions

☐ Seeking medical tests that were not recommended by a medical professional

☐ Independently seeking alternative treatments that were not directly suggested by your provider (e.g., naturopathy)

☐ Consulting friends or family who are healthcare providers (instead of your treating providers)

☐ Texting your doctor/medical provider

☐ Calling your doctor excessively

☐ Calling to get earlier appointments with medical providers

☐ Sending unsolicited photos in electronic medical records or in emails to your doctor

Cyberchondria

☐ Internet searches about physical symptoms or conditions

☐ Internet searches about possible treatments or treatment alternatives

☐ Excessively researching possible side effects of medications or procedures

☐ Joining, following, or seeking online forums for those with unexplained medical symptoms

☐ Selectively researching or seeking out personal stories of negative health outcomes to justify excessive health seeking behavior

☐ Frequently reading or watching the news (which tends to sensationalize and lure people into watching with negatively biased portrayals and language regarding health outcomes)

Self-checking
- ☐ Excessive mirror or physical body checking (e.g., searching for bumps/blemishes)
- ☐ Excessive mental "check-ins" of body sensations or physiology (e.g., heart rate, breathing)
- ☐ Palpating (touching/pressing) body parts or repeatedly moving limbs or head to see if one can feel a problem
- ☐ Excessive weighing of oneself
- ☐ Taking blood pressure or pulse readings/wearing technology that takes physiological readings such as a Fitbit or Apple Watch
- ☐ Taking your vitals using blood pressure cuff, pulse oximeter, or other tool
- ☐ Wearing unnecessary medical alert bracelets

Excessive Preventative Behaviors
- ☐ Being overly rigid about sleep (e.g., overly precise bedtimes/wake times, trying to "catch up" on sleep after a night of rough sleep, avoiding staying up later)
- ☐ Overuse or rigid use of vitamins/supplements
- ☐ Changes in your diet and exercise routines, or overly restrictive diets
- ☐ Excessive handwashing or sanitizing
- ☐ Telling others what precautions to take (e.g., having others wash or sanitize before entering your home, forwarding recall notifications)
- ☐ Making unneeded doctor's appointments ahead of time "just in case"
- ☐ Always keeping EpiPens or other fast-acting medication close by without doctor's instructions to do so
- ☐ Making sure you always have safety items with you, such as a charged phone, water bottle, etc.

Other Health Behaviors
- ☐ Writing down symptoms prior to doctor visits
- ☐ Bringing/sending excessive records to doctor visits

☐ Checking your medical records and interpreting them without speaking to your physician for clarification or interpretation

☐ Preparing for catastrophe when is it is not imminent (e.g., writing a will, saying goodbye to family members, planning who will take over your work)

☐ Superstitious behaviors to protect health (e.g., not breathing in when you pass a cemetery, not saying the word "cancer" in same sentence as mentioning a loved one)

Avoidance

☐ Avoiding doctor or dentist visits

☐ Avoiding taking routine medications or important procedures that are suggested by a doctor

☐ Avoiding saying or hearing words related to themes such as medicine, health, or death

☐ Excessive avoidance of people that "look sick" or were recently sick

☐ Avoiding buildings that are reminders of health content (e.g., walking past or inside medical buildings, hospitals)

☐ Insisting that others avoid talking about medical content around you

☐ Avoiding media, television shows, or movies that show medical content

☐ Avoiding driving past cemeteries

☐ Avoiding going to funerals

☐ Avoiding scheduling or doing activities during times that you are waiting for medical test results or when you are feeling anxious

☐ Avoiding things that lead to normal physical sensations (e.g., riding as a passenger in a car over hills, hot or muggy locations, amusement park rides, spicy foods)

☐ Researching restaurants or new foods before eating them; or avoiding new foods

☐ Refraining from strenuous exercise (when not directed by a doctor) or movements you fear would worsen symptoms

Mental Review

- ☐ Rumination/excessively trying to mentally figure out "what to do" in response to symptoms
- ☐ Excessive body-scanning (i.e., repeated mental "checking in" to see if you feel OK)
- ☐ Overly trying to figure out what might be the cause of symptoms

Other

- ☐ Any other excessive health-related behaviors not mentioned above:

_____

_____

_____

Gaining Awareness by Monitoring Anxious Responses

Now that you have identified some of your excessive approach and avoidance behaviors, we can start to learn and practice behaviors that will reduce your anxiety in the long run. This generally means reducing avoidance of anxiety triggers, and gradually reducing overprotective behaviors. To begin to develop a plan of attack, we will have you self-monitor your anxious behaviors using a template that is very similar to the one you completed earlier in this workbook. This time, we will also ask you to examine how you responded—what you did (or did not do) in response when you noticed your anxiety. This will help us gather some information on just how frequently these behaviors are occurring and the types of situations or thoughts that may be driving these behaviors. See the next page for an example log. We encourage you to keep this log for at least one or two weeks so that you get enough information to formulate a plan to attack these behaviors, which we will discuss next.

Anxiety Response Monitoring Form (Example)

Trigger (thought or situation)	Anxiety level (0–10)	Response (approach or avoidance strategy)—what did you do in response?
I noticed my heart beating faster while cooking dinner. I had the thought, "I might be having a heart attack."	8	I talked to my partner and asked what I should do. He said I was fine, but I was not sure and I told him I wanted call an ambulance instead. I laid down to avoid exerting myself.
I noticed a strange sharp pain in my arm that I haven't noticed before. I had the thought, "I might have cancer."	6	I researched "sudden arm muscle pain" and related terms online to see what it might be. I then ruminated about the pain for the rest of the day.
My friend mentioned that she went to her annual medical exam with her doctor. I had the thought, "I haven't been to the doctor in years."	4	I changed the topic and avoided scheduling a routine appointment.
My mom started talking about her bloodwork results.	9	I started crying and demanded that she stop talking about medical stuff.

Anxiety Response Monitoring Form

Trigger (thought or situation)	Anxiety level (0–10)	Response (approach or avoidance strategy)

The Vicious Cycle of Anxious Behaviors

Now that you are gaining some more awareness of your triggers, fears, and behavioral responses to fear (excessive approach or avoidance), let's talk a bit about why these behaviors seem to persist even though people often suspect they may not be helpful in many ways.

First and foremost, exaggerated health-related worries provoke anxiety! If you are telling yourself negative thoughts like "This might be a heart attack that could kill me on the spot," you are likely to feel very distressed! When people are anxious, they tend to try and get control of or reduce anxiety and uncertainty in some way, usually via behavioral responses—trying to do something to lighten the anxiety associated with these thoughts. They begin to use avoidance or overprotective behaviors to get a sense of control. We do this when anxious because it can work quite well in the short term—we might get a brief, relieving sense of control. However, these behaviors are exactly what keep health anxiety going in the long run, as we get quite addicted to them and never learn that things continue to be OK even when we don't rely on them.

It makes sense and is normal to avoid things that are dangerous, but in the case of health-related anxiety, the relief that is offered by these responses is only temporary and can negatively impact daily life functioning. Avoidance often serves to reinforce fears that uncomfortable thoughts are correct, and that the anxiety and doubt associated with them are intolerable. Further, over time, the behavioral responses often get more appealing and the urge to use them becomes stronger, thus requiring more and more not-so-adaptive behaviors in order to feel that brief sense of security. This problematic cycle is depicted in Figure 3.1, and an example of an anxious situation applied to the cycle is depicted in Figure 3.2.

Over time, the avoidant response may provide temporary relief from anxiety, but also serves to keep the fear alive. The person depicted in the example cycle in Figure 3.2 may conclude that they are not able to hear about others discussing their medical

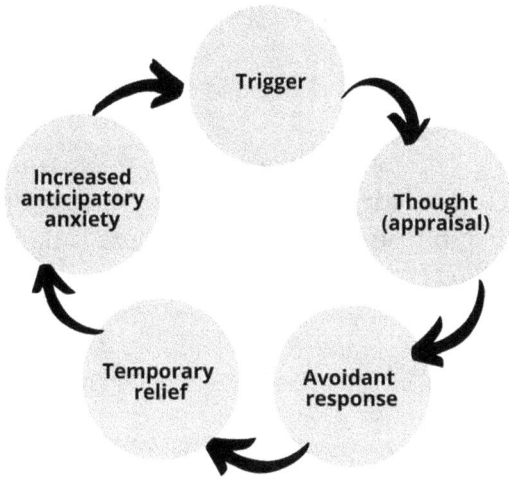

FIGURE 3.1 Illness anxiety cycle

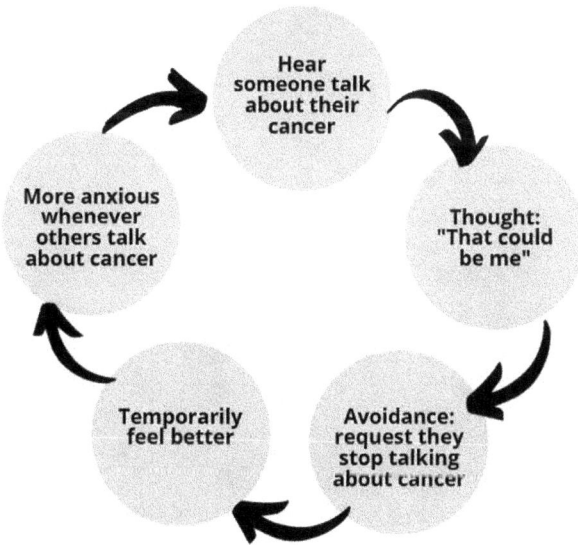

FIGURE 3.2 Example of IA cycle

conditions, and that anxiety is intolerable. They would not have a chance to learn that they could handle it on their own, that they could tolerate the uncertainty, and that their fear of developing cancer would not stay high if they did not use excessive avoidance behaviors.

Therefore, approaching fears and reducing protection from them is critical to reducing health anxiety. In the next chapter, we will discuss how to begin to approach some of these fears in a gradual way that should feel manageable.

4

How Your Thinking Perpetuates Health Anxiety

Common Health Myths

While you are spending a couple weeks monitoring your anxious behaviors using the Anxiety Monitoring Form in the previous chapter, let's talk a little about anxious thoughts and how they impact health anxiety. When people are excessively anxious or depressed, they tend to think in ways that maintain or contribute to their feeling that way. Often they do this without even being aware of it. If we can begin to identify and be aware of these thinking patterns, we can notice them and challenge them. If the anxious thoughts are leading to undue distress, we can change them. You may feel that thoughts happen to you without your control. This is true to some degree, since our brains and bodies are not always controllable. But you do have quite a bit of control over what you pay attention to in any given situation, how much you believe the thought or feeling you are having, and how much you engage with it. The first stage in reducing anxious thinking involves just increasing awareness that these anxiety-increasing thinking patterns are happening. These anxious thoughts and feelings are often not literal phrases we are saying to ourselves in our head, but rather outcomes that we are implying to ourselves may happen. However, when we are

DOI: 10.4324/9781032711355-4

anxious, these thought patterns and predictions we are implying are often biased and incorrect. Thinking in these ways tends to make us feel worse. To begin to identify if some of these thoughts are relevant for you, we have listed some common beliefs that tend to show up in illness anxiety. We call these health myths because they are often believed or felt strongly, despite a lack of concrete evidence that they are true. Not all of them may apply to you, but we often find that many or most of them likely will. Carefully consider whether you have ever thought in these ways, and write your detailed responses in the blanks provided.

Myth 1: Any Physical Symptom Means I Am Dying or Have an Undiagnosed Medical Condition

The most common thought pattern related to illness anxiety is noticing a physical sign or symptom and catastrophizing about it—thinking it is a sign of something to be concerned about. If you have illness anxiety, keep in mind that you are very likely to overly interpret routine and benign physical symptoms as signs of serious illness. Do you think that sounds like you? Take a moment to think carefully about the following questions, and write your responses in the blanks:

What physical sensations have you been alarmed about over the past several weeks?

_____

_____

_____

What did you tell yourself about these symptoms? What medical issue, if any, did you tell yourself a symptom may be a sign of?

_____

_____

_____

How often were you right in your predictions? What eventually happened?

_____

_____

_____

Your interpretation of your bodily sensations is likely to be quite biased: it is often highly influenced by recent things you have heard or experienced, stories you have heard about from the media, and how your family/social circle tends to respond to signs of illness. In addition, often we are inadvertently seeking information that will selectively confirm what we expect to hear, whether it's doing biased internet searches, asking other health-anxious family members for advice, seeking doctors who we think will be able to give us reassurance or more certainty, and so on.

Related to this health myth is another thought that often goes something like, "It's always best to catch things early." Individuals with illness anxiety are often overly attentive to their own bodies, fearing that if issues are not detected early, disaster will ensue. We can acknowledge that we have often seen commercials and other media with the message, "Early detection is key." While some aspects of this way of thinking may certainly be accurate, do you see any potential problems with constantly approaching health in this way? If yes, write them below:

_____

_____

_____

Healthy Bodies Are Noisy Bodies

One potential problem with the above thought pattern is that benign physical sensations are a routine occurrence for most people. Even the healthiest of individuals will experience benign but unusual and/or uncomfortable physical sensations on a daily or weekly basis. Often they are not noticed as much by healthy individuals, because the average person does not consider them meaningful. People with illness anxiety are more likely to notice and catastrophize about routine bodily symptoms that others may ignore or tolerate.[1, 2] People with illness anxiety view body sensations as signs of poor health, while people without illness anxiety are more likely to view many bodily sensations as normal and expected even in a healthy body.[14]

If you can remember a time before you had health anxiety, you may think that you did not often have physical sensations, and lament the fact that you now do! However, it is likely that you also had weird sensations then as well. You may not have noticed them at the time as they didn't have the same scary meaning for you. Rather, they were routine physical sensations that didn't need to be explained, and weren't considered to be signs of serious potential illness. Hyper-focus on physical sensations can also distort and magnify the size and scope of the sensation. You've probably had the experience where you've stared very closely at an everyday word and it starts to look strange over time. A similar experience happens when we pay too close attention to our own physical sensations: they become distorted and amplified over time as we scrutinize them.

Below, write down an example of a time when you had symptoms that your medical providers were unsure of the exact cause of:

_____

_____

_____

What was the outcome? Was it helpful for you to try and determine the cause of the sensations, or did it result in more anxiety? In retrospect, how concerning was this symptom?

_____

_____

_____

Myth 2: Every Symptom Is Explainable

As mentioned above, individuals with illness anxiety are likely to think that nearly every physical symptom is meaningful. Not only that, they often think that such symptoms *should* be explainable, in that a cause should be identifiable. They may also take it a step further and think that every symptom should be able to be tested for and able to be identified by medical professionals, and sometimes even believe that almost everything should be treatable.

This thinking style can lead us to forever be on the "chase" for the right explanation and treatment. It is important to practice tolerating uncertainty related to not always getting a straightforward diagnosis and/or treatment plan from your doctor, as this is quite common in medicine. Over your life, how many times have you (or someone you know) been to visit a medical provider and the provider gave you several potential explanations for your symptoms? Indeed, quite a bit of medical care is educated guesswork. When you are not provided with the exact root of your problem and/or a solution, how do you feel when you leave the doctor's office? Likely, you feel confused or frustrated at the lack of palpable outcome and certainty. However, we need to recognize that even experts have limitations and do not always know the answers. Sometimes they should not know the answer and be able to acknowledge when they do not.

The reality of it is that most bodily sensations cannot be explained in the moment. Certainly, there are causes of the sensations, but often it is not things we can readily identify or know for certain, and searching for a cause can get quite futile. Often. the cause(s) of sensations are very complex due to several factors such as sleep, mood, diet, temperature, or other factors. Just because a sensation is unexplainable to us does not mean that it is dangerous or meaningful.

Myth 3: I Can't Trust Doctors; I Can Only Trust Myself

A common belief among people with illness anxiety is that medical providers are not adequately doing their job. Individuals with illness anxiety may feel unheard and misunderstood by doctors, or feel a need for health reassurance that is just not met by speaking with doctors. It is not uncommon for patients to report to us that they feel like doctors minimize their complaints, do not spend enough time with them, overlook their concerns, or even treat them with apathy, dismissiveness, or criticism. As a result, they often overwhelm their medical providers with information—sharing every possible sign and symptom that may be meaningful, hoping that the doctor will be able to assemble this complicated puzzle if only they as a patient provide the right information. Often, our anxious patients can cite times when they and/or someone they know had a bad experience with a physician or other medical provider, or cite times they felt their personal research or excessive hunting of the answer was the one thing that really saved them from medical disaster.

I do take [parents of patients] seriously and listen. It won't work to have a dismissive demeanor or take a very short time. Taking them seriously and giving them my undivided attention and listening to all of what they want to say even if they have lots of symptoms. I often bring in my own kids or experience, e.g., 'my daughter had a cold for three weeks,' and validate that they are worried about their children. I may point out to them if they keep coming in for the same thing. Often there's something deeper underlying the more exaggerated than normal response, like some story of a cousin who died after a fever. I take complaints seriously and try to be attuned to what is going on in the entire family; parents may have anxiety themselves. It's stupid to keep seeing the same person for the same thing and not addressing what is happening, which is, the parent is nervous.

Dr. L., Pediatrician

Certainly, not every physician is an excellent physician, and even the authors of this book can recall some visits with physicians after which we are left wondering how this person possibly could have graduated from medical school. However, often people with illness anxiety are basing their feeling of dissatisfaction on their feeling of unease in leaving the doctor's office, and usually this unease comes from not having a clear answer to the medical question. As mentioned in Myth 2 above, not every symptom is readily explainable or meaningful.

Almost always patients with illness anxiety report that they feel that they must advocate for themselves, do their own research, and plan their own healthcare, lest serious health conditions be overlooked by a careless doctor. It's rare to work with someone who is not able to point to at least one story in which they feel that their health research or self-advocacy saved them from a missed diagnosis or treatment.

First, yes, let's absolutely acknowledge that doctors are human, and therefore are certainly fallible. They make mistakes, just like all humans do. They also have significant time and attention pressures on them that may add to the chances of making mistakes. However, this does not necessarily mean that they do not care, that they weren't cautious, or that you can never trust another doctor and must take things into your own hands to prevent death and disaster. Also, simply because they have made mistakes does not mean that they are ineffective and their advice should be ignored, overridden, or aggressively supervised.

Remember that you have biases in your thinking such that you are more likely to notice and remember things that are consistent with your fears. This means that you are more likely to recall times when you feel like your protective behaviors were helpful, and less likely to recognize and remember all the times when they did not lead to anything productive. Also, it is unlikely that you experiment with not using protective behaviors very often, which prevents you from realizing that usually the outcome is the same when they are not used.

I see the gamut of anxiety, whether it's patients or family. Someone might come into the [inpatient] unit, we rule out things like a stroke, then it's time to go home, and they might be hesitant. Whether it's the patient or family member, they think that because the patient is in the hospital that that's where everything is available and it's the best place to get any kind of care. So we sometimes run into family or patients that were expecting more: they were expecting answers to every single problem. Sometimes it's obvious that it's actually that family member that's super anxious or depressed.

Dr. L., Internal Medicine

As an example, a past patient of mine told me about how strongly she felt that her own medical research and knowledge was helping her stay safe. She came into one session feeling stressed, but somewhat victorious that she had identified her own medical issue. She noted that the radiologist had done a recent routine ultrasound of her breast and had told her that she needed a biopsy, and to schedule this biopsy at her earliest convenience. The patient reported that she immediately became anxious and spent five or six hours calling around to try and find a medical center that could get her in within a week to complete a biopsy, as she didn't want the anxiety of the looming test hanging over her head during the week. She reported that the entire weekend after scheduling the appointment she engaged in much internet research about the biopsy, and in doing so discovered that because of a pre-existing health condition, she might not need to do the biopsy. She noted that she then contacted all her doctors (which were numerous) to try and have them share records to better communicate. She then contacted the referring doctor and convinced him that the biopsy was not necessary, based on her research. She noted feeling indignant and frustrated when her primary care doctor finally acknowledged that the biopsy was not necessary, and noted that she felt she had saved herself from an extra test. Surely the radiologist was inattentive to her chart, and she would have been sent for an unneeded biopsy without her own intervention! This reinforced her belief that she must scan her own body, do her own research, and advocate for herself, lest something serious be missed. Makes sense, right?

Take a moment to think about her approach. Certainly, there are some merits, but what are the costs? She spent almost an entire weekend engaging in health-related research, feeling extremely anxious. She called around to rush the test when such urgency was not requested by the doctor, potentially preventing her healthcare providers from having adequate time to review the recommendation and her records. Once her primary doctor was informed of the appointment, her doctors may have eventually cross-referenced and informed her that the test might not be needed. The most pernicious part about this is that it reinforced the idea that she needs to take her own healthcare into her hands. She was prevented from learning that if she does not take such cautionary steps, she will still turn out OK. In the end her actions led to ongoing hypervigilance as she continued to scan herself for additional problems and press her doctors in similar ways.

We do want to encourage you to be appropriately informed about your medical conditions if you have chronic medical issues or diagnosed conditions. We encourage you to ask your doctors for advice about these conditions and even research these conditions if necessary to help guide you in how to best cope with them. However, this can cross the line into people trying to become their own doctor. There is a reason it takes seven to ten years to become a doctor! So how might you know when you are excessively trying to be your own doctor? This may be occurring if you are doing any of the following:

◆ Researching health-related topics you probably already know the answer about, or have already researched

◆ Seeking new treatments or tests that your doctors have not brought up with you

◆ Managing your own care (e.g., discontinuing medications or prescribed treatments) without consulting the prescriber

◆ Avoiding things that your doctor has not directly instructed you to avoid—e.g., exercise, driving, caffeine

◆ Avoiding taking medications or doing treatment that your
   doctor has prescribed without informing the prescriber
◆ Seeking several second opinions or new healthcare
   providers
◆ Having too many healthcare providers

These are just some examples. Is there anything else you can
think of that you do/have done when trying to play the role of
"doctor"? If yes, write it below:

_____

How much do you think it has reduced your worry about health
in the long term? Could you prove in court with evidence that
this behavior alone was what saved you, or were there other factors that may have contributed? If yes, list those potential factors
below:

_____

_____

_____

How do you think your doctor feels about this behavior? Do you
think they would approve? If not, what do you think they would
recommend?

_____

_____

Myth 4: If a Doctor Wants to Rule a Disease Out, That Means I Likely Have That Disease

Over many years as clinical psychologists, we have discussed
and witnessed numerous medical concerns among our patients.
Annual visits to a primary care physician commonly result in
"flagging" potential issues for further testing and/or discovering
legitimate medical concerns that may need to be addressed. For

example, a diagnosis of an enlarged thyroid upon physical examination may require further diagnostics, such as a sonogram. Test results such as breast lumps or abnormal blood work are very common and frequently result in additional testing, such as may result in your doctor suggesting biopsies, more blood panels, additional mammograms, and so on. Periods of testing can involve long intervals between appointments and feedback, and require us to sit with much uncertainty. Because of this, the interval between the physical examination and further diagnostics is a prime time for anxiety to amplify and the "What if ...?" questions to flourish. For example, "What if ... they find something, if I have cancer, or I die?"

If your medical provider suggests ruling out a problem with additional testing or exploration, remember that does not mean that you have the problem; it does not even mean that it is likely. The medical system, at least in the USA where the authors are located, is still a business. Therefore, healthcare organizations still very much care about patient satisfaction, and generally want to avoid complaints, claims of malpractice, and repeat contacts from anxious patients who eat up their time. For this and other reasons, many healthcare providers will tend to err on the side of caution and request testing to rule out possibilities. This is another reason why we suggest that people generally avoid seeking second opinions or multiple care providers unless directly recommended by a medical provider—usually more providers means more testing and more questions. In addition, doctors will often order additional testing just to appease the patient (especially if that patient is known to be an anxious client!), even if the doctor wouldn't have pursued such testing if they were in the same scenario.

Additional testing is commonplace. Therefore, you will have times in life when you will need to wait for the results of important medical testing. Remember, how you think and behave during these times can either keep your anxiety manageable, or escalate it. Base your thinking on what you believe: what is the most likely outcome—rather than rare outcomes that could occur. If scary outcomes are likely, you can plan for them appropriately. However, they are usually not the most likely scenario. Behaviorally, continue life as usual, and accept that there will be some uncertainty and anxiety in your day to day living. It's OK to have some appropriate worry! Expecting yourself to not be anxious about things tends to cause more discomfort.

As a final note, just because a doctor has mentioned potential diagnostic labels for your issue does not mean that they have formally diagnosed that issue. When the doctor says, "It could be MS (multiple sclerosis)," an anxious person might hear "You have MS," rather than what the doctor is trying to say, which is, "There is a rare chance it could be MS." Because anxiety craves certainty and order, we grasp and cling to diagnostic labels to get a sense of control and understanding. However, many diagnoses are provisional, which means that they are possibilities to be ruled out. In addition, just because a doctor has given you a diagnostic label, it does not mean what you are experiencing is a medical *problem*. Diagnoses are labels used to communicate information; and while they are most used to describe pathological conditions, you cannot assume they are necessarily indicators of disease or need for intervention. Doctors frequently provide diagnostic labels for issues that are benign and do not warrant attention or treatment. These scientific labels can sound scary, but at times they can be describing things that aren't typically cause for great concern. For example, "dysplastic nevi," or "tonsillolith," and "herpes simplex 1" can sound scary, but are technical names for benign irregular moles, tonsil stones, and cold sores, respectively—diagnoses that are generally considered quite common and relatively uneventful bodily disturbances. We have seen many of our patients get alarmed when they hear labels such as these! The takeaway message from all of this is to be careful about how you interpret medical labels— just because something has a label or scientific-sounding name does not mean that it is a medical condition that warrants concern and attention. Ask your doctor for clarification if you are unsure, rather than making assumptions and being your own doctor.

Magical Thinking and Thought-action Fusion

One error in logic that we sometimes see related to Myth 4 is what is sometimes called "thought-action fusion." What this term means is that sometimes we have a strong sense that how we feel or think has an impact on reality, in almost a magical or superstitious way. You may or may not have this type of thinking associated with your health anxiety, and the strength of how much confidence we have that our thoughts influence reality can vary. For example, some people may feel strongly that if they talk about a health outcome, or if someone mentions a scary thought or event, that will make the outcome more likely. "Magical thinking" occurs when we begin to make associations that aren't causally linked in the real world. For example, a person who got food poisoning after watching a movie may avoid watching that movie ever again, for fear they will get sick again if they watch it. As the movie can't possibly transmit food poisoning, they have made an erroneous inference that the movie somehow led to their illness. Much of the time, people are aware of the illogical nature of the connection and how it doesn't fully compute, but still feel it's too scary to take the risk. These superstitious-type feelings are common to obsessive-compulsive disorder, but can also show up in other anxiety disorders such as illness anxiety.

Do you have this sense that your thoughts might impact the world around you? If yes, take a moment to examine that feeling: do you feel you can influence only negative things and not positive ones—that is, can you use your mind to influence the universe such that you win the lottery? If not, what does that tell you? If your thoughts could influence reality, why doesn't it work for good things as well as bad? Anxiety can trick us into believing the mere presence of a thought means the outcome of the thought is more likely to happen.

An example we frequently use to test this out with patients who obey this strong feeling is to have them focus on an airplane flying in the sky. Together we look up at that airplane and say out loud, "I want that plane to fall out of the sky, I want people to fall to their deaths." Even people without anxiety disorders will likely experience a surprising level of anxiety when saying this statement. When the people do not fall out of the sky to their deaths or the plane does not crash, your slowly start to learn that you may not be magically capable of taking down a plane with your thoughts. This example demonstrates how strong feelings do not always match up with the evidence available to us, and that feelings are important, but should be taken with a grain of salt as they are often wrong!

Myth 5: My Health Risk Is Different, So the Normal Rules Don't Apply to Me

Sometimes health-anxious people have good insight into their anxiety. They may be aware that the medical issues they are afraid of are rare and unlikely. They may be aware that others would not be as concerned and would not protect themselves as much from these catastrophes. However, they may say something like, "But my health is fragile," "Bad stuff seems to happen to me more than others," with the implication that somehow the rules don't apply to them and they need to be extra careful.

Again, it's certainly possible that you may have struggled more with health issues than most people, and/or that it often seems like you are getting ill frequently. It may even seem that you have bad luck and bad things just seem to happen to you more often than others. However, maybe we can step back and take a closer look at this feeling while factoring in the thinking biases that we tend to have when anxious. Individuals with health anxiety tend to report that they think their health is worse than others who have the same medical conditions.[14] Often, people feel they experience more than their fair share, and they are often basing it on a subjective sense rather than evidence. They often cite times that they have gotten ill when others hadn't, or list off all the medical issues they have had over their life.

How much do you believe that what you are experiencing is outside the norm of what people typically experience? What are you basing this on? Could you prove in court that you are more likely to have these medical conditions than other people? With what evidence?

Some people might say yes to this, and if that is the case for you, some realistic problem-solving around health might be necessary to make sure that you are taking *appropriate* measures to take care of your health and prevent negative outcomes. However, most people with Illness anxiety acknowledge that they have special rules they follow to take care of their health that they are aware an average person might not follow. Take a moment to think about this—are there any things you do to monitor, test, check in on your health, or to prevent health outcomes, that you think an average person might not do (and that your doctor has not recommended)? If so, list them below. This will likely be useful to know when you are developing a plan to tackle anxious behaviors in a later chapter.

My "special" health guidelines:

_____

_____

_____

_____

_____

_____

Finally, commonly the things that people with illness anxiety are doing to try and prevent health disaster backfire and may make them paradoxically more likely to experience health issues. For example, they may be handwashing excessively, or using antibiotic medication prematurely and/or frequently. Some exposure to germs is recommended, as your immune system relies on this to develop and be resilient. Overuse of antibiotics tends to breed antibiotic-resistant strains of bacteria that are harder to treat in the long run.[3, 4] Or you may be seeking opinions form several doctors, which as we noted above, tends to lead to more testing, questions, and different opinions that are hard to reconcile, rather than the certainty or clarity you were hoping for. Trying to avoid every physical symptom leads to feeling constantly attentive to physical symptoms, and to feeling that these things cannot be tolerated, increasing pain and discomfort over time.

In short, is important to weigh the costs and benefits of your health behaviors. Are you doing what an average person might do in that situation? If not, why not? What about you is so special that the rules just don't apply?

Myth 6: Because It Could Happen, I Should Try to Do Whatever I Can to Prevent It

We often hear people say something like, "Yes, I know it's unlikely! But I just can't tolerate the possibility that it can happen, no matter how small." They justify their hours spent in trying to prevent the feared medical catastrophe by saying that because such an outcome is possible, efforts should be made to prevent it. However, do you see any problems with that way of thinking and behaving?

If this seems to apply to you, first take a moment to consider whether you think this way just about health, or broadly, in many areas of your life. Do you generally follow a life philosophy of, "Because [negative thing] is possible, I should do whatever I can to prevent it?" Do you drive a car? Do exercise as much as you should? Do you neglect checking your smoke alarm regularly and do you mindfully limit fire hazards in the home? Do you own firearms? Do you use alcohol? All of these things are risk behaviors as well, and associated with many preventable deaths each year, yet most people with illness anxiety are falling short on carefully doing protective behaviors for at least some things like this, because we have gotten used to them, don't view the time and effort as worth the risk it mitigates, and/or don't view them as terrifying as medical illness. Typically, health-anxious people are taking risks in some areas but not others, despite a potentially higher risk of death or injury in those other areas. In illness anxiety, your excessive focus becomes your health, and you can ignore the positive ways you are already tolerating distress in your life.

As this book is being written, heart disease remains the leading cause of preventable death in the United States,[5] as it has been for several years. Do you exercise several times a week, avoid fats and sugars and eat your vegetables daily, and avoid other cardiac risk factors such as smoking? If not, don't worry—you are like most people! These recommendations are hard to keep up with at all times. However, if you truly wanted to invest in limiting your risk of health issues developing, the reality of it is developing some moderate heart-healthy behaviors is a great way to start. What we are trying to convey is the fact that often people are sitting around worrying about rarer catastrophic health issues that may pop up, are engaging in selective health behaviors that "put fires out," and they are not doing basic self-care behaviors that could more realistically reduce risk in the long term.

You would think, given that people with illness anxiety are extremely conscious of their health and use medical services more often,[6, 7] that this increased engagement would lead to at least a *little* bit of improved health, given the time, money, and mental effort invested! However, research suggests that the health behaviors people with illness anxiety tend to engage in are not related to better health outcomes than everyone else. All of the checking, reassurance, research, and so on are not related to how many illnesses people have across their life,[8] and how likely they are to develop a serious illness.[9]

Some people have a broad life philosophy of trying their best to prevent negative outcomes, even ones that have a very small chance of occurring. They are generally hypervigilant to threats of many kinds, and feel very threatened by anything that is out of their control. Health issues are obviously one of those areas—the unfortunate reality is that sudden and unexpected health issues do happen sometimes, and while we can do some things to reduce risk and improve outcomes, we simply cannot control health outcomes in many cases. It's important to examine what you are doing to try and control your health to ensure that it is worth it in the cost-benefit analysis, which we will discuss in detail below.

Myth 7: My Extreme Health Vigilance Is Necessary to Prevent Catastrophe

Now, you might be one of those people who is on board with all the myths we described above, and may even be able to see them in your own thoughts and be aware that they are distorted and tend to make you feel worse. You may be able to realize that your excessive health behaviors are exhausting and perpetuate the cycle of anxiety. At this point, despite good insight, some people still have a hard time letting go of their excessive worry and rumination about health. You may feel that your worry is the only thing that keeps you vigilant and ready. If you think about stopping your health worry, right this minute (regardless of whether you can do that or not), does the idea of not worrying concern you, even a little? It's not unusual for people to have a strong feeling that if they stop worrying, they will miss something—that is, not detect an important symptom in time for it to be treated, or will become lazy and unaware of their own body, or some other problematic consequence. This feeling can stop them from disengaging from the rumination cycle at times when they might be able to, and when it might be helpful to do so as it is not leading to additional productive action or problem-solving.

If you are afraid of dropping the worry rope, let's examine this idea a bit. We already mentioned in the previous section that individuals with illness anxiety are not less likely than anyone else to develop serious medical issues, suggesting that their health behaviors and mental vigilance don't lead to significantly better health outcomes. In addition, much research suggests that extra doctors' visits are more likely to lead to testing that is at best unnecessary, and at worst possibly iatrogenic, or harmful.[10, 11] The research also suggests that people with illness anxiety are actually *less* likely to follow through on behaviors that are correlated with good health, such as following doctor's recommendations and regular good hygiene habits.[12] Individuals with illness anxiety are more likely to have their physical symptoms (or worry about symptoms) interfere with their life: they are more likely to miss days of work, and more likely to rely on disability benefits, even more so than medical samples who do not have illness anxiety.[9] How much do you believe your worry is helping you?

Beliefs about the Value of Worry

Sometimes people have a sense that their worry might be helpful, at least in part. These beliefs can often be hard to identify.

When we ask people, "Can you think of any pros to your worrying?", most people say, "No way! I hate worrying!" Yet they have a hard time giving it up, even when they can look at the evidence and say that their worries are quite irrational based on the available evidence. This is often because even though excessive worry backfires on people and there are many downsides, there are good sides as well. We tend not to do things repeatedly unless there is something rewarding about them that keeps them going.

To a large extent, worry is a behavior. What we mean by that is that it is to some degree a choice. Worry at its core is your brain problem-solving, trying to find an effective approach, such as trying to brainstorm alternatives for what you might do in a particular situation, or think through the situation in way that you feel may prevent you from being caught off guard or disappointed should your feared outcomes arise. It is, at its core, a productive thing, in that it helps us plan for negative things in the future—which is why we do it! It helped keep our ancestors alive to plan for potential dangers. However, it easily gets out of hand if you are excessively preparing for danger, and/or you find yourself on a worry hamster wheel: you are thinking about the same things over and over again without any conclusions about productive actions you can take.

Also, even if there are moments in which your brain gets carried away and you find it wholly uncontrollable, you can still decide how much attention you give the worry voice, and how you respond to it. Intrusive worry can be a lot like a bully that follows you around: the bully may try to poke you by constantly reminding you, "You should be scared about this! Don't you *care* about this potential danger?!" But as loud or annoying as the bully tries to be, you can still decide whether you are going to listen to it and let it get you worked up, or whether you will keep doing what you are doing and let the bully talk. Just like real bullies, the more you tend to turn to the worry and engage with it, trying to argue with it, giving it your time and attention, listening to it, the more it will bother you and escalate over time. If you ignore the bully and simply let it say what it wants to say, it will fade away just like a bully who loses interest. You can step back from the voice and decide what you personally, according to your values, want to do in the situation.

However, because worry can be functional at times, people sometimes have beliefs about what will happen if they do not worry about health. These concerns can prevent us from giving up worry or relaxing our vigilance, even if we can recognize that it might help us feel better. Because these can be hard to identify, let's review a few examples so you can think if any of these might be the case for you.

"Worry Prevents Me from Feeling Disappointed or Taken Off Guard"

Individuals with health anxiety often feel that their worry is preparing them for the worst in some way, and that if they were to stop worrying, they will be unready for disaster, and as a result even more upset should their feared outcomes occur.

Doing a Cost-benefit Analysis of How Much Your Worry is Helping You

If the above sounds like you, it is certainly possible that some worrying in advance helps prepare you to some degree—again, that's why humans do it at all—but take a moment to think about whether it has been worth it for you, in a cost-benefit analysis. Maybe we can do it a bit right now. Can you think of a few relatively recent episodes of strong worry about your health? Fill out the chart below as thoroughly as possible. There's an example entry to give you a sense of what it might look like.

Cost-benefit Analysis of Health Worry Worksheet

Health anxiety episode (what I was worried about and when)	How much of the time did I worry? For how long?	How did the worry help you think of any beneficial approaches or help you be more prepared? How sure do you feel the worry was required?	Was the benefit worth the costs of worry?
I read in my report that the doctor had labeled my past cancer "metastatic." I had such strong worry that this meant it was likely to come back, even though I am in remission.	Worry at an extreme level, most of each day, for around five months!	The worry may have helped me slightly in reminding me to ask my doctor about it, as I didn't realize what it really meant. Otherwise, I don't think it helped me think of any new or helpful courses of action.	No! The amount of benefit I got was minimal, with high cost.

For most people, in doing this chart they will see that the benefits of anxiety often do not outweigh the high costs of worry. While there certainly can be pros of worry, as it does sometimes help us feel more prepared, when it is excessive we tend to run around in circles in our head without a lot of productive problem-solving.

Most people with illness anxiety find that they are worrying in advance to try and prepare for things that never ever happen.

This is certainly an odd strategy: make yourself feel miserable in advance so that you feel less miserable eventually? Some preparation in advance is warranted if the outcome is quite likely and there is an aspect of effective problem-solving that can be done. For example, a patient of mine was worried that her cancer (which was now in remission, but had a fairly high chance of recurring, according to her doctor) would return, and that she would have to go through treatment again. The treatment caused significant problems the first time around when she had not anticipated financial and childcare burdens of going through such a rigorous course of treatment. In that case, some level of measured problem-solving in advance may be appropriate, discussing among the family who may care for the children if the patient is temporarily unable to work or has medical appointments. However, remember what we have been saying all along about anxious thinking: when people are anxious, they tend to over-estimate how likely and how scary things will be. Therefore, their "planning" is often inaccurate, as they are planning for a situation that even it if it occurs, is often little like what they imagined.

There are times in which we feel our worry was helpful, in that it did help us prepare or result in us taking some productive action. In that way, worry is very reinforcing and keeps itself going. These episodes can stay fresh in our mind, and we may cite them as reasons for continuing to make sure we worry enough. However, we may forget about all the times that we worried and nothing happened. This is why the cost-benefit chart is important to ensure you carefully weigh whether the pros that you are getting from worrying about your health are worth all the cons.

"If I Don't Worry, Scary Outcomes Are More Likely to Happen"

Usually, this type of thought or feeling is a form of magical thinking—a type of thinking we described earlier in this chapter. Magical thinking is a strong sense that our thoughts or feelings have an impact on the world around us. Most people can recognize that this seems a bit irrational—but still may have a strong almost superstitious feeling that it could be true. This magical thinking is a normal feeling in most people—even people without anxiety disorders tend to have some discomfort if they say things aloud such as, "I wish my mom would get cancer!" Even though we can recognize that science suggests saying such a thing aloud would be unlikely to change the actual likelihood of our mom getting cancer, for most people it is still hard to do! Magical thinking can relate to hesitancy to drop the worry hope at times. For example, sometimes people have a sense that they must do a sort of penance by worrying about bad events. They may have a feeling that if they worry and suffer about something enough, this will prevent the powers that be from delivering this scary outcome.

If this sounds like you, take a moment to think about whether you actually believe you can impact your surroundings with your thoughts or feelings, or whether this is simply based on a feeling. Most people recognize that it's strongly based on a feeling and they wouldn't testify in court that it is fact. If you experience this strong feeling, we highly suggest doing relevant exposures. In a later section, we specifically detail how to do exposures that are designed to test out magical thinking kinds of feelings. If you feel that you will be punished by some higher power if you do not worry, this can also be tested through exposure and behavioral experiments. Also, think about what you believe: do you believe in a higher power? If so, according to your personal beliefs or religious teachings, does it make sense that the higher power would punish you for not worrying? Why and how would this happen? Many people can recognize that, based on their system of religious faith, there is no logical reason why they would be expected to worry about their health excessively. If you are unsure, and have a religious leader, you may want to consult them about what your faith says about whether your god would want you to suffer with worry about your health. You may want to make sure you speak with a religious leader who is familiar with health anxiety, obsessive-compulsive disorder, and/or anxiety in general. They can provide a realistic grounding of your faith and complement what we are covering in this book.

5

Designing Your Exposure Hierarchy

Hopefully now you have started to take your anxious thoughts with a grain of salt. Next, let's begin to talk about changing your behaviors to get more evidence to convince your brain that your anxious feelings are often inaccurate.

Approaching Health Fears

Learning to approach fears, rather than shying away from them, is arguably the most important part of cognitive behavioral treatment for anxiety and related issues. The method for learning to approach feared content is called "exposure," and it is used in treatment for nearly all anxiety disorders. The word and concept of exposure may sound intimidating, but what we mean is that we must face fears in order to overcome them. We tend to do this in a gradual fashion, starting with things that are barely challenging to you, practicing that situation/feeling/experience over and over, and then moving on to progressively more challenging situations until we reach the most difficult things that you are avoiding. By the time we get to the most difficult, it will not feel as daunting as it did at the beginning. It's like a Jenga tower that starts to get shorter the more you take the pieces out from underneath. You are likely familiar with this concept just from

DOI: 10.4324/9781032711355-5

your personal experience—usually people can think of things that they originally thought were frightening, but did them over and over, and realized that it wasn't so scary, such as learning to swim or ride a bike, or taking your very first rides on a roller-coaster. In doing these things, we gradually approach our fears and learn that we will be OK, and that while the situation feels scary, we can handle it.

The concept of exposure is generally easier to demonstrate for simpler fears, so let's use an unrelated fear as an example: fear of dogs. When people come into our clinic for treatment of a phobia, such as fear of dogs, we gradually have them face their fears. They are always in control, and choose each exposure exercise they do, but the goal is to take progressive steps to get used to feared situations. So they might start by doing something like just looking at cartoon dogs or photos of dogs, and then practice that until it does not cause discomfort. Then the patient may start by walking past dogs that are fenced-in, and slowly approaching but not touching them. Then they may finally encounter a small dog, and at the end maybe spend time in a room with larger dogs. They generally end up doing something it was hard to imagine doing at the start of treatment, but after taking several successive steps, it no longer seemed so unmanageable. You can actually start to enjoy part of the experience, and develop confidence in yourself along the way.

We use this system of exposure to treat illness anxiety fears as well. The exposures are tailored to people's specific fears, but as an example, someone who avoids hearing about cancer may start by just talking about their own cancer fears, then may move on to reading information about cancer, and then practice hearing others talk about their own personal experiences with cancer, then attend cancer screening visits (e.g., mammograms) that they have been putting off.

As you are likely just starting to work on your anxiety, you may think that it's hard to imagine ever being able to confront some very anxiety-provoking situations. That is totally normal! As exposure tends to work up a ladder—starting with mildly challenging things to confront and working its way up, by the time you get to the things that are most fearful for you, they should seem more tolerable. You will likely have done so much that you will be more used to those anxious cues, and more likely to realize that your feared outcomes are unlikely to occur in the way you are imagining.

A primary goal of exposure is getting evidence to test feared outcomes. Therefore, when possible, the first goal of exposure is to test whether your feared outcome occurs or not (remember that anxiety makes it seem that negative outcomes are more common than they actually are). Second, given that you are likely also making predictions about how bad the situation will be, we also want to test how you handled the situation (i.e., Did you lose control? Was the anxiety as intense as you thought it would be? Did it stay at a high level, or decrease with time, etc.). In exposure, we are trying to retrain the body to accurately assess threat, and thereby decrease anxiety over time.

The first time you practice an exposure, you may feel a fair degree of anxiety, as you are facing your fears. Over time, if you stay in the situation and allow the body to experience the anxiety (thoughts and physical sensation) without trying to control it or escape, the anxiety will subside naturally. As you repeat the exposure practice, you will get a chance to see whether your feared outcome occurs and will learn to assess more accurately how dangerous a situation truly is. The more you practice exposure, the less fear the situation and accompanying anxiety feeling will elicit.

Some people at this point will ask, "But I've done this [exposure situation] so many times, and I never get more used to it. Why am I still scared of it?" In response, we often take a close look at their past experiences with the feared situations, looking closely to see if there were any subtle avoidance or attempts to control anxiety. When people are encountering their feared cues and not getting more used to them, more subtle avoidance and control strategies typically are typically being used. For example, they may be going to previously avoided doctors' appointments, but bringing a loved one with them in case they get too anxious. In this way, they are confronting the anxious situation, but not fully. They are still doing mild protective behaviors. Therefore, the brain learns, "I was OK, but only because I relied on [subtle protective behavior]." You will be unlikely to fully habituate (i.e., get used to a situation) until you relinquish all of your protective behaviors. Sometimes the protective behaviors can be very subtle and/or mental, such not looking in the direction of a feared thing, or excessively reassuring yourself there will be no serious mental diagnosis. The truth is that you cannot know for sure that you will not receive a serious medical diagnosis, although it is likely a slim chance. Exposures involve walking towards this uncertainty mentally and with your actions. We know it is difficult to be in the moment and fully face your fear when engaging in the exposure, but as soon as you notice your mind is drifting, whether to a neutral part of the room or to more anxious thoughts, it is of the utmost important to bring your full attention back to the exposure at hand.

Exposure therapy has been a core part of anxiety treatment for decades, and has been shown to be very effective in improving symptoms of most anxiety disorders, including illness anxiety and related issues.[1-5] It is arguably the most effective and proven ingredient of treatment for anxiety. Most of the research on exposure suggests that it works by changing people's anxious beliefs about their feared situations.[6-8] That is, when people do experiments to test out their feared predictions (such as "I can't tolerate this," "This will last forever," or "If I do not check this I will end up in the hospital," etc.), they often find that their fears are disconfirmed in several ways. Typically, people find that their feared outcomes do not occur at all! However, sometimes some aspects of feared outcomes do occur. In these instances, people may also find that some elements of their anxious predictions are disconfirmed—for example, they may find that they were able to tolerate the situation much better than they anticipated, or the outcome did not play out in as catastrophic fashion as they had imagined. For example, a person who predicts that they will catch a serious disease and end up in the emergency room where they are not cared for appropriately and die as a result may find instead that they do get ill, but they recover quickly, that the doctors were more receptive than anticipated, and were able to treat them effectively.

While exposure seem to change people's thoughts for the better, we often find out from patients in treatment that they are
doing the opposite: they are waiting for their thoughts to change
prior to confronting anxious situations! That is, they are often
hoping that we as therapists can make these avoided situations
less challenging and anxiety-inducing before they enter them.
They often think that there must be a way we can somehow "talk"
them into feeling less anxiety before they must face anxious situations. In fact, it works the opposite way, in that changing behaviors changes your anxious thoughts. One must first take steps
towards anxious situations for thoughts about it to change and
become more adaptive. They do not have to be big steps right at
the get-go, but waiting around for the situation to get less anxiety-provoking typically is not productive or feasible. One of the
most important things people can learn from exposure work is
that they can tolerate anxiety[22, 24] and choose how they want to
behave, no matter how anxious they are. Your brain will also
learn that while anxiety can be strong, it is not always accurate,
and that it will go away with time without anxious behaviors—
it cannot last forever. Unfortunately, however, our brains don't
seem to "learn" this until we actually *do*—we can talk about
these feared outcomes and challenge them, but we find that most
of the change happens when people behaviorally test them and
see the evidence for themselves. For example, if I am someone
who is generally apprehensive about riding rollercoasters, someone could explain to me all the reasons why rollercoasters are
actually safe and all the inspections and safety statistics that are
out there to protect rollercoaster riders, but I am still going to
feel afraid of getting on the ride myself until I have done it a
few times. I logically know the safety data, but I am unlikely to
feel the learning physically until I have done it myself. Most of
the time, our behavior must change first to notice a difference in
our feelings and beliefs. We realize this requires a leap of faith,
which is why most people confront exposures gradually (but not
so gradually that they do not take risks!).

There are multiple forms of exposure that may be helpful for you to try. Designing your own exposure exercises can feel difficult, so we will provide several examples and tips. Generally, creation of an exposure ladder starts with rating situations you are avoiding or overprotecting yourself from. You can get a sense of these from the Health Behaviors Checklist you completed in Chapter 3. If you are willing, and have people in your life who can provide honest feedback, it can also be helpful to ask people who know you well—family or friends—what anxious behaviors they have noticed you do. Sometimes loved ones who know us well can pick up on things we weren't even aware we were doing—or weren't aware were unusual. Sometimes loved ones are also compensating for our anxiety in their own lives and interactions with us as well, which is another form of protective behavior.

Now that you have completed the Health Behaviors Checklist and have self-monitored your anxiety for at least a week or two, you should have a decent sense of how you are thinking and behaving when it comes to your anxious situations. To start drawing up your exposure hierarchy, let's first re-inventory your anxious cues. In the list below, write down the situations you are avoiding due to anxiety (e.g., hospitals, people who talk about health, health-related TV shows, etc.). We have listed a couple examples to show you what it might look like. Make sure to do a thoughtful, through inventory, reviewing your checklist and self-monitoring if necessary.

My Avoidance List

People, places, things, sensations/feelings, or thoughts I am avoiding because of anxiety or fear:

Example 1)	Entering hospitals (I could get sick from the germs there)
Example 2)	Watching medical drama television shows
Example 3)	Making dental check-up appointments (they could tell me something is wrong)
1)	
2)	
3)	
4)	
5)	
6)	
7)	
8)	
9)	
10)	
11)	
12)	
13)	
14)	
15)	

In the second list below, write down all the health-related behaviors you are doing that you have identified may be excessive. As described in previous chapters, these anxious responses may take several forms: avoidance of feared situations or cues, excessive reassurance seeking or body checking, or even mental activities such as excessive mental problem-solving or trying to replace bad thoughts with good ones, etc.

In the second column, list how often and for how long you are doing these behaviors. In the final column, write how often you think an average person might do these behaviors. If you are truly unsure how often others may engage in these behaviors, before proceeding stop and do some research—ask several others who are not anxious about health how often they do this behavior and for how long to get a sense of what might be "average." We suggest you refrain from consulting the internet!

My Health Safety Behaviors List (Example)

	Health-related safety behaviors I am doing	On average, how often and for how long I am doing this behavior?	My estimate of what a typical person does
1)	When I notice a weird new sensation, asking my husband if I should call the doctor (I know he will say it's up to me)	Every time I have a weird new sensation, around twice per month. I ask him one or two questions each time.	They might ask their spouse twice per year, and only if they do not know the answer themselves already!
2)	Washing my hands excessively	10–15 times per day, for around 90 seconds each time.	I know the guidelines are to wash for around 60 seconds. Most people probably wash only 5–10 times per day, and use only one, not two pumps of soap.
3)	Checking my blood pressure daily (my doctor has not directly told me to do this)	Once every morning	Several of my family members said they'd do this only if a doctor has recommended it, and do it as often as they instruct.

My Health Safety Behaviors List

	Health-related safety behaviors I am doing	On average, how often and for how long I am doing this behavior?	My estimate of what a typical person does
1)			
2)			
3)			
4)			
5)			

Creating Your Exposure Hierarchy

Now you should have a thorough list of situations that you are likely avoiding due to anxiety, and safety behaviors that you do to try and reduce or control your anxiety. These lists will be the foundation for creation of your exposure hierarchy, so you may want to return to them to make sure you have done a very careful inventory before proceeding.

The next step is to create an exposure hierarchy, or ladder. You do not have to include all the situations you listed above. Examine the first list you made of situations you avoid. While you may be able to arrange exposures to all of these situations, and in some cases that may be appropriate, it is often easiest to start with ones you want to be able to do, or do with more ease. Which of the situations you wrote down do you wish you could do, or do with less anxiety? In the exposure hierarchy form in the following table, write down the situations you have identified that you are avoiding due to health anxiety, that you want to be able to do. Exposure hierarchies should be detailed and step by step. If one exposure feels much higher than the step below, then try to think of exposures in between that should be on your list. This is where we need you to put on your creative thinking cap. Get as creative as you can. Sometimes creating different iterations of exposures, combining different permutations of exposures to thoughts, feelings, situations, experiences, and/or people can provide nice interim exposures between bigger steps on the ladder.

Once that is finished, write down the situations you identified that you are avoiding which an average person may encounter in their routine life experience. For example, most people can attend doctor's appointments, get blood draws/vaccines, take medications that are prescribed, walk into hospitals, touch commonly used objects without washing hands immediately after, and so on.

Next, review the other list you made, the Health Safety Behaviors List. On the exposure hierarchy form in the following table, write down the estimated frequency/duration/type of this behavior that you suspected most people may do. For example, if you take five preventative vitamins, but suspect that most people take none, you might list something like "stop taking vitamins unless prescribed by a doctor" as a potential exposure item.

An example list so far may look like the following. In this case, to demonstrate the inclusion of both avoidance and safety behaviors, the avoidance behaviors are the first three listed, and the next three are safety behaviors the patient wants to reduce.

Potential exposures	Anticipated SUDS (0–100)
Enter hospitals	
Watch medical drama television shows	
Make dental check-up appointment	
Ask spouse for reassurance about medical issues/symptoms no more than twice per year, and only if I truly do not know what their answer would be	
Handwash for no more than 60 seconds, no more than 5–10 times per day, and use only one, not two pumps of soap	
Take my blood pressure at home only if a doctor has recommended it, and do it as often as they instruct	

Now, next to the behavior in the final column, you will be asked to make a rating of how anxious that situation would be for you if you were placed into it or asked to confront it *right now*. This rating should be based on how anxious or uncomfortable you would be if you were forced to endure this situation without protective behaviors or avoidance. To rate, we typically use a 100-point scale that has commonly been used in previous anxiety disorders treatment and research, called the Subjective Units of Distress Scale, or SUDS, which is depicted below.

SUDS Scale

Please rate your level of anticipated distress on a scale from 0–10 (or 0–100):

0	25	50	75	100
No problem	*Discomfort noticeable to you (but you could hide it if you wanted)*	*Moderate but manageable (you are uncomfortable, but can still do things)*	*So anxious I have uncontrollable physical symptoms that are/ would be noticeable to others (e.g., trembling, turning red, sweating, etc.)*	*Worst ever*

Using this scale, estimate how uncomfortable you would be in each situation, or if it is a safety behavior, how uncomfortable you would be if you reduced it or ceased it entirely. Write your rating next to the exposure task on the right side in the SUDS column. You can use any number between 0 and 100; you do not have to use 25-point increments, those are just reference points to give people some anchor points for rating. (Other programs or clinicians may use different indicators for this scale, but we have found that these anchor points can helpful in providing esti-mates.) Note that it should be rare that you give a 100 rating! A 100 rating, or close to it, should be reserved for the absolute worst anxiety you have had—so theoretically, this should be reserved for the one most difficult scenario.

Now look at your ratings, and how many exposure situa-tions you have listed. Sometimes people list too few or too many exposure situations. Typically, we recommend around ten items, ranging from 30 to 100 in SUDS rating, and having around five to ten points in between. If you find that all your situations are highly rated, or there is otherwise a large gap in ratings some-where in your ladder, it is likely possible that you can break down one of the higher-rated items into an easier step or set of steps to "bridge" the gap. If you have rated two things similarly, you may want to remove one of them to make your hierarchy smaller. Below is an example of what a final exposure hierarchy may look like for our example person:

My exposure hierarchy (example)	Anticipated SUDS (0–100)
Take my blood pressure at home only if a doctor has recommended it, and do it only as often as they instruct	30
Watch medical drama television shows	35
Read about people's personal experiences of coping with serious health issues	40
Handwash for no more than 60 seconds, no more than 5–10 times per day, and use only one, not two pumps of soap	48
Ask spouse for reassurance about a health-related issue less than once per week	55
Ask spouse for reassurance about medical issues/symptoms no more than twice per year, and only if I truly do not know what their answer would be	65
Walk around the outside of a hospital (but do not go in yet)	70
Walk around the inside of a hospital	75
Make and attend my child's dental check-up appointment	85
Make and attend my personal doctor check-up appointment(s)	95

My exposure hierarchy	Anticipated SUDS (0–100)

A Note about Cyberchondria

One of the most common health-related behaviors that we see is cyberchondria, or using the internet to research health or engage in unnecessary health-related activities. Maybe you have experienced how easy it is to get sucked down an online hole in which you end up doing way more health-related research than anticipated? Most people report that they tend to feel worse after this activity, or that it led to some very brief relief, with anxiety worsening in the long run. Research suggests higher use of the internet to research medical questions is related to worse illness anxiety in the long term.[9-11] Research suggests online health research to be a particularly pernicious cycle of anxiety-driven searching, a brief sense of relief, but more researching and more anxiety in the long run.[11] The nature of the online world of information—abundant, but varying in quality and accuracy—pairs with anxious traits such as perfectionism and intolerance uncertainty to create a perfect storm of escalating anxiety.

> *The right answers and the wrong answers are all out there [on the internet]. I say, 'Show me what you are looking at.' We have resources at the hospital that provide us with up-to-date information. The problem is when [patients] still believe what they read even though you've told them it's not really a site that can be trusted, or other sites that suggest it's different. For example, I recently had a patient insist that an antidepressant medication dose be 200 mg as she saw it online, but it was for a different diagnosis, and the 20 mg dose was an appropriate starting dose. She was receptive and realized that it wasn't as simple as Googling it. Unfortunately, there are bad outcomes that happen; there are doctors who don't take the time to explain things correctly or make mistakes. Because of that there is a decent amount of self-imposed advocacy. So these experiences validate patients, but unfortunately also gives them more juice: 'I really got to stay on top of this stuff.'*
>
> *—Dr. L., Internal Medicine*

These searches typically start out with good intentions, and the intent of being knowledgeable is not necessarily a bad thing—we want you to be educated! However, the searching can become rigid, lengthy, urgent, and confusing. Excessive internet searches often lead to one hearing about catastrophic outcomes that are possible, but highly unlikely. Given that conflicting data and many individual opinions are out there, they can end in a great deal of confusion as one tries to reconcile all the varying opinions. Occasionally, people come across some tidbit of information that makes them feel better temporarily. That is why this behavior keeps going: it is intermittently reinforced as it leads to some brief relief. However, in the long run it leads to people feeling more confused and anxious as they get information overload and feel that they need to keep researching to be safe.

As you may know, as you use the internet, much of your searches and activity are entered into constantly updating computer algorithms that are designed to feed you more content related to what you appear to be interested in. Therefore, unfortunately, the more you research about catastrophic health outcomes, the more likely you are to be shown them in online ads and suggested content. For example, a person who is repeatedly researching symptoms of cancer and potential cancer treatments online may soon find that they are seeing more online content related to cancer—making it seem like cancer is everywhere!

Because internet research can be so pervasive and tempting in health anxiety, and is so likely to increase anxiety in the long run, we suggest that everyone with illness anxiety limit internet research or online health-related activities (such as visiting message boards regarding health). We encourage you to work these activities into your exposure hierarchy. If you feel that going cold turkey in giving up all internet research is too hard, you may want to start with setting some limits about when you will use the internet regarding health issues. Some people then make progressive steps on their exposure hierarchy in which they reduce the use over time. If you choose to do this, as with most exposure items, we encourage you to be very specific about under what circumstances you will or will not use the internet. You may also want to practice delaying your research for progressively longer stretches of time, as most people with illness anxiety have a sense of urgency to their searching—when they get a symptom or issue, they need to know now!—and have trouble waiting and sitting with uncertainty. To give you an idea of what this tapering off internet use may look like, an example person's cyberchondria-related hierarchy items may be as follows:

Limit health research to 30 minutes/week, use a stopwatch	50
Limit health research to 10 minutes/day, use a stopwatch	65
Wait 48 hours before doing any health research	75
Entirely refrain from health-related internet research	95

Exposures Related to Magical Thinking

In Chapter 4, we noted that sometimes people with illness anxiety experience what we call "magical thinking." Again, magical thinking occurs when we feel that our thoughts or feelings have an impact on the world around us despite generally knowing that our thoughts cannot control or impact others. For example, we may feel that if we think a lot about illness, or if we say things about our health out loud, or think negatively in general, that makes those outcomes more likely to happen. Sometimes people report that they feel that they need to worry about their health in order to do some kind of penance—and have a feeling that if they do not worry "sufficiently" about their health, they will be more likely to be struck by a health disaster. Sometimes people are even avoiding saying certain health conditions aloud, or mentioning the names of loved ones as they talk about these conditions, feeling it will be more likely to happen if they talk about it.

Do you think any of this sounds like you? Do you think your thoughts might have some impact on reality? If so, the good news is that it is relatively easy to design exposures to challenge magical thinking, and if you are experiencing magical thinking, we highly suggest that you add these types of exposures into your hierarchy.

To do this, take a moment to consider what you truly believe, versus what you feel to be true. Often what people truly believe—that is, what they would believe "on paper" or would testify as true in a court of law—is different from what they feel. Do you truly believe (i.e., would testify in court) that if you do not worry about health, a health disaster will ensue? Or that if you talk about a disastrous health outcome, it will be more likely to happen? If so, how would this work? In your understanding, what deity or force would lead to this happening? Why would this happen, in your opinion—for example, if you are religious, why would a god want to punish a person for not worrying about their health? According to your belief system, why would this happen?

Most people recognize that they do not truly believe that their thoughts or statements make health outcomes more likely. After all, if such a phenomenon works in a negative direction, couldn't it also work in a positive direction? If thoughts impact reality, wouldn't we be able to think ourselves into good health?

If you do not truly *believe* that your thoughts impact reality, but continue to *feel* worried that they might, this is an excellent opportunity for exposure. To do this, include exposure items designed to test out the power your thoughts may have. For example, if you fear that thinking about cancer will make it more likely you get cancer, then you may decide to do an exposure to make it a point to sit and think about cancer for at least 20 minutes each day. If you think that discussing diabetes out loud makes it more likely you will get it, then practice saying diabetes-related words aloud for 30 minutes each day. Better yet, challenge your superstitious feelings by making or writing statements such as "I hope I get cancer" or "I would love to die of cancer." Feels wrong, right? But that is the point of the exercise, to illustrate that just because we feel something strongly does not mean that it is true or accurate. Collect some evidence about whether your thoughts impact reality by doing testable experiments in which you try to think or talk yourself into certain outcomes—good or bad.

Tips for Refining Your Exposure Hierarchy

Take Reasonable Risks

For the most part, try to design exposures that are reasonably safe, that most people would at least be willing to try, and are not known to cause harm in large numbers. Early exposures are typically things that you are aware you are avoiding that you may not need to be avoiding. Middle exposures tend to be things that most people encounter in life without avoidance. Final exposures tend to be "overlearning" exposures, in which we really try to test fears by doing things that people might not encounter on a routine basis. Since designing these overlearning exposures can be complicated, we discuss this in more detail in a section below.

Don't Get Hung up on the SUDS Rating

If you are having difficulty rating your situations, or the process of trying to rate and order them is causing you too much grief, don't sweat it. Sometimes people can be too perfectionist about the hierarchy of exposures. Doing each step on a gradual ladder of exposures is also not a requirement. If you feel you are confident you can jump to a higher exposure sooner and endure that situation without protective behaviors, then by all means go for it! However, make sure you feel reasonably confident you can stick it out without avoidance or protective behaviors, to avoid doing these behaviors and having the exposure backfire and reinforce avoidance. It certainly happens sometimes that we underestimate how difficult a particular exposure will be, and once in it, find that it was way more difficult than anticipated. If you feel severe, incapacitating anxiety during an exposure, it's likely good to take a slight step back—make the exposure slightly easier so that it is still challenging but doable, returning to the full exposure after practicing the modified step until it is less anxiety-provoking.

The Exposure You Are Working on at the Moment Should Be Challenging but Doable

An exposure exercise is unlikely to be effective if does not push you out of your comfort zone and create some discomfort. We often find that patients play it too careful and sometimes go too gradually over time, not taking enough risk. This leads to their experiencing discomfort for longer periods of time and being in treatment for much longer periods than necessary, and preventing them from learning that they can feel uncertain and still survive. The goal is to be gradual, but also to take some risks. Do not be afraid to list situations on your exposure hierarchy that you can't even imagine yourself trying to do at the moment! It is expected that exposures will help things get easier gradually. By the time you are doing exposures at the top of your hierarchy, you will have done so much practice that at that point it should seem much more doable.

The Best Exposures Are Designed to Directly Test Your Anxious Predictions

The best exposures are ones that use a scientific experiment to directly test your anxious fears. This is not always possible, but in many cases it is. Many health-anxious predictions are testable. Some examples are:

> *"I cannot tolerate hearing other people talk about their health—I will be anxious for days after."*
> *"I will get sick if I enter a hospital."*
> *"If I attend my doctor's visit, I will get news the cancer is back."*

In these cases, direct scientific experiments can be engineered to test whether these outcomes are true and as bad as people are imagining, or whether the anxiety is talking!

However, with many worries related to health anxiety, the predictions are so far in advance that they are not testable any time soon. Alternatively, our feared outcome may have many potential causes, and we can never be sure what factors may have contributed. Some examples are:

> *"If I get Hepatitis, I will not be able to enjoy life"* (too far in future to test, and may not happen)
> *"I will get cancer if I don't take these vitamins"* (too far in the future and not testable, as if you get cancer, we cannot be sure what the cause is)

While these certainly reflect worries that are exaggerated just like other health anxious worries, they are not immediately testable. In these cases, we can do imaginal exposures, which we describe in a section below.

Your exposures should confront things you are avoiding because you are trying to avoid or control anxiety. Often people lose sight of the point of the exposure and think the point of an exposure is to make themselves miserable and to sit in discomfort as much as possible. In our opinion, you do not need to delve into things to intentionally frighten yourself if it is not something you would avoid due to anxiety. For example, some of our well-intentioned patients would come into session and tell us that they spent several hours reading catastrophic news stories about people who suddenly died of rare health conditions, or read about several medical conditions in detail. These are fine exposures for someone who would avoid this material when they encountered it due to anxiety, or someone who needs to confront it (e.g., a nurse who needs to be able to hear others talk about health issues). In those cases, we would generally only suggest they persist with it until they habituate. However, for others who aren't avoiding it or will need to encounter it in routine life, it is likely that reading awful news that just makes you sad (rather than anxious) just reinforces distress. Sometimes it is better to refrain from seeking out biased negative sources such as the general news which provide overly negative and sensational takes. Exposures can be uncomfortable at times, but the goal of exposures is not to make yourself miserable, but rather to test your fears, and to ensure that you can do things without avoidance when you need to. If you can do these situations already without notable anxiety or avoidance behaviors, you likely do not need to pursue them further.

Make Sure to Be Accountable in Keeping to Your Exposure Schedule

There are many ways to do accomplish this goal. We sometimes expect that as adults, we do not need reinforcement, but in fact, we naturally include it in our everyday life. For example, after a busy five-day work week, do you continue working all weekend, or do you treat yourself to a movie, reading a book, spending time with family and friends? You reward yourself with participation in these activities because you know by the time Monday comes around and the work week begins, you will need to feel replenished. Well, the same concept applies with keeping to the exposure schedule. We encourage you to be compassionate with yourself, accepting of anxiety, but also accountable for doing the regular exposure exercises knowing that they are critical for improving anxiety.

For some individuals, the plan to stay accountable is not enough. We encourage you to think over whether you want to include a loved one or someone from your social support network to help keep you accountable in continuing with your exposures. This person should be supportive, non-judgmental, and very encouraging. If you do not complete an exposure or fall behind, let them know the positive ways they can help you get back on course rather than any shaming approach. You want to be comfortable working on the same team towards the same goals together.

Practice Often, and in Many Different Situations

Most formal treatment programs for anxiety that use exposure suggest that people complete exposure daily. Sometimes these programs do several hours of planned exposures daily if the anxiety is severe. We do find that there is a good relationship between the amount of exposure work people do and how much improvement in anxiety they report. Therefore, we encourage people to do at least 30 minutes of planned exposure a day. By planned exposure, we mean setting aside formal time to specifically confront the next item on your exposure hierarchy. Many people make the error of trying to wait until they "run into" situations and don't plan out exposure time or try to seek out exposure opportunities. For example, a patient may return to session one week and say, "I didn't practice tolerating unusual physical sensations because I didn't have any." Subsequent exposures may then be designed to create prolonged periods of unusual new sensations and practice tolerating them. Or someone may say, "I didn't do an exposure of listening to others talk about health issues because none of my family or friends talked about health this week." We would then encourage them to seek out things they are avoiding rather than passively waiting for them—for example, specifically asking others about their health issues, or doing an internet search for videos of other people discussing their personal experiences with medical issues.

Seeking out exposures, rather than just waiting for them to come to you, often adds an important layer to the exposures:

voluntarily seeking out and choosing to an exposure that was not necessary in daily life can test fears that are related to an overestimated sense of responsibility. For example, someone may fear that by touching many items in public settings, such as touching doorknobs, railings, and public pens without washing or decontaminating, may lead to increased chances of catching a serious virus. While touching the few public doorknobs that they come across in a week is certainly great practice, the best exposure would be to touch many different railings, doorknobs, and public items daily for long periods of time. For many people, having to seek out "extra" exposure to these things (i.e., beyond what they might encounter in daily life) adds an element of risk and anxiety that is important to practice tolerating as well. Usually, these fears are related to scary feelings of responsibility: that you chose to take on additional risk, even though you didn't have to. Taking these risks can help you learn that taking some acceptable risks does not always lead to catastrophe.

Time spent doing exposures is important, but it is also important to conduct exposures in several different situations when possible. This is to ensure that you generalize—that you become less afraid of these types of situations across the board, rather than just under those specific circumstances. For example, if someone only practices tolerating weird physical sensations at home, they may get more used to them at home, but be thrown by them when they occur out in public.

Plan to Stay in the Situation for a Prolonged Time When Possible

Related to the above comment about time spent doing exposures, we recommend that you do exposures for a prolonged period, staying in that situation without avoidance behaviors. It's not always possible to stay in the anxiety-inducing situation, but when you can, it's typically best to stay in the situation rather than doing brief exposures only. For example, watching videos of others talking about their health conditions (if that is one of your exposures) for several hours is likely to be much more helpful than watching a single two-minute video. Or for those who avoid entering hospitals, taking 35 minutes to do a detailed walk through a hospital is better than going into the lobby for a moment and then leaving. The bottom line is that the more that you are exposed to that situation without using safety behaviors, the better chance you will have to disconfirm your fears. A person who is worried that they will get sick from germs in a hospital will be unlikely to learn that their feared outcomes are unlikely if they simply enter the hospital and then move on. However, if they stay there for a very long time, touching several surfaces and encountering people, this is likely to give much more data to suggest that they can survive such experiences. Try to remain in the exposure as long as possible, but at least until your SUDS decreases by half.

Refrain from Safety Behaviors When Possible

Any exposure is likely to be less helpful if you engage in safety behaviors. Safety behaviors, as described above, are smaller or subtle forms of avoidance that prevent people from fully confronting their fears. An example of a safety behavior might be handwashing excessively after you are in a hospital, or asking someone if your mouth looks swollen after you eat something you feel you might have suddenly developed an allergy to (despite no history of allergy). As mentioned above, sometimes people may already be entering feared situations, but have not been getting more used to them over time; we typically find that this is because they are continuing to rely on safety behaviors in these scenarios. Sometimes they can be very subtle and hard to detect. They can also be mental: for example, someone who enters a feared situation (e.g., a doctor's office), but refuses to look at or think about the real cue that makes them anxious, such as the crowds of people who are touching the same items they used and potentially transmitting germs. A tip is that with most exposures, you should notice your fear level decrease at least a little over time. If after an hour of direct exposure you are not noticing even a slight reduction in anxiety, it is likely that you are not confronting what makes you anxious about the situation, or using some sort of safety behavior. To catch this, ask yourself, "Is there anything I am doing right now to try to reduce the anxiety associated with this experience, or to try and prevent my feared outcome?" Sometimes we will engage in hidden safety behaviors and it is difficult to discover what is happening and why our anxiety is not decreasing.

As we mentioned in the "Creating Your Exposure Hierarchy" section above, stopping all safety behaviors abruptly may be too difficult if you are engaging in many of them. Therefore, you may need to plan tapering them off as part of your exposure plan. In these plans, the person would limit factors such as who they would seek reassurance from, the number of times they could ask, or the amount of time they could spend on internet research per day or week, or about what kinds of things they could ask or research. The idea is to reduce the behaviors gradually but fairly quickly.

Starting Exposures

As homework this week, look at your exposure hierarchy and choose an item to start with. Most people start with a situation that is around 30 SUDS—only slightly challenging. Ideally, you should practice this situation every day (or as much as possible), and stay in that situation for at least 30 minutes a day. You are unlikely to test your feared outcomes sufficiently unless you gather a large amount of data that is convincing to your brain! Otherwise, your brain is likely to explain away these successful encounters as "flukes" that happened by accident. Remember to try to minimize or not use any safety behaviors (things you do to protect yourself from anxiety), such as asking others for reassurance or excessively trying to convince yourself you are OK.

Use the chart below to track your predictions and SUDS ratings over time as you do your exposures. Before you do the exposure, write down your estimated SUDS rating and anxious predictions on the Exposure Tracking Form below. There is an example completed form to demonstrate what it might look like. Completing this form every week as you do exposures and keeping a record of them is an important way to scientifically test your anxious predictions. It's also often a helpful record to have and review in the future if you notice your anxiety kicking up again!

Designing Your Exposure Hierarchy ◆ 123

Exposure Tracking Form (Example)

This week's exposure:

From now on, take my blood pressure at home only if a doctor has recommended it, and do it only as often as they instruct.

Anticipated discomfort (SUDS)	My anxious predictions: What do I think will happen when I do this (e.g., will I get hurt, ill, or die)? How uncomfortable will I be, and for how long?	Actual SUDS the final time I did the task this week	Actual outcome
30	For this one, I am aware the risk is low. I do not think I will die or miss something critical. I think I will just think about it constantly for the rest of the day.	20	I was anxious for about 15 minutes after I had the urge to check my blood pressure, then I usually did something else and forgot about it. It was also slightly less anxiety-provoking and easier to do than I thought.

My Exposure Tracking Form

This week's exposure:

Anticipated discomfort (SUDS)	My anxious predictions: What do I think will happen when I do this (e.g., will I get hurt, ill, or die)? How uncomfortable will I be and for how long?	Actual SUDS the final time I did the task this week	Actual outcome

Here we reiterate the importance of doing the exposure work to the successfulness of improving illness anxiety. Often, people think that they can simply read through the materials in this workbook without completing the written exercises or doing the real behavioral work of the exposures. We view that as being like a person who wants to get in shape, but goes to the gym and only reads about how to exercise! Certainly, we want you to be informed, and reading about your anxiety can certainly sometimes be helpful in planning. But changing illness anxiety requires investment in behavioral change. And just like that person in the gym, to truly "get in shape," daily exercises are required.

If you are still having problem identifying what might be a good exposure for you, that's OK. Exposures are different for everyone, since everyone has different fears related to health. However, if you need to get your brain jogging or are still having a hard time identifying what things you may be avoiding, below are some actual exposures that our patients have done, to give you some examples. Keep in mind that the best exposure for you will be a situation in which you are avoiding or using protective behaviors that others likely do not use as much, and one in which you can test your fears and get some concrete evidence (through experience) as to whether your anxious fears are correct or not. If it is something you are not avoiding and does not cause you at least a bit of discomfort, you can move on!

If you give yourself a good chance and find that you are still are having trouble developing your hierarchy or starting exposures, you may want to seek help from a professional therapist who can help give you more guidance. It can be easy to be hard on yourself for having difficulty with exposures, but they are challenging! It is not uncommon for people to feel like they need additional support during this time. We encourage you to be compassionate with yourself and seek help from loved ones or a qualified therapist if you are feeling stuck.

List of Some Example Exposures
Reducing Avoidance

- Scheduling a routine doctor's or dentist appointment
- Scheduling and/or attending routine testing, bloodwork, or checkups your care providers have recommended
- Watching a video clip from a fictional medical television show
- Watching videos/clips about people's personal experiences with serious illness (e.g., cancer)
- Watching video clips about doctors giving "bad news"
- Reading about the treatment process for the serious illness(es) you are afraid of
- Reading about an unsolved medical scenario
- Taking a medication as prescribed
- Not avoiding discussing health when others need/want to discuss their health conditions
- Reading books about death/dying or chronic illness, such as *Being Mortal* by Atul Gawande or *When Breath Becomes Air* by Paul Kalanithi
- Visiting friends at a hospital, or going to a hospital
- Not asking friends to change their topic of conversations if they bring up a frightening topic

Decreasing Health Behaviors
Usually, these exposures involve reducing or completely refraining from body checking related to health (that has not directly been recommended by a doctor), such as:

- Refraining from taking your temperature at home
- Refraining from use of blood pressure cuffs, pulse oximeters, thermometers, or smartwatches that enable you to check your heart rate, temperature, or blood pressure
- Stopping body checking, such as pushing, pinching, scanning yourself in the mirror or for health signs
- No longer weighing yourself at home (e.g., get rid of scales)

- Refraining from making lists of symptoms to bring to your doctor or journaling medical symptoms
- Reduce or discontinue taking over-the-counter supplements or vitamins
- Discontinue looking at ingredients
- Do not talk about health with others unless they ask you direct questions about it, and do not ask questions for reassurance

Refraining from Asking Others about Your Symptoms
- Refraining from online medical research
- Making sure all appointments are recommended by and referred to by your GP (i.e., use your GP as a gatekeeper for all other providers, rather than seeking out your own specialists)

A Note about Using the Internet for Exposures
You probably noticed in the above list that watching videos with health content online or using the internet to research health-related issues can often be a great way to do exposures. However, some people are hesitant or confused about how to use the internet for exposures, as we have often told them it's best to avoid perusing health-related information on the internet to reduce cyberchondria! So why would we now have you go back into it?

The internet is full of information, and is where most people get their information these days. We do not expect you to never use the internet for health-related information. We also want you to be informed, and we view moderated education about health conditions and appropriate preventative behaviors as healthy.

Controlled exposures to health-related videos or searches on the internet can be very helpful (a) if you are avoiding this content due to excessive anxiety, and (b) if you do so in a controlled, unbiased way. First, there is generally no need to seek information online or do exposures to health videos if you would not be avoidant of this content in the first place. Second, one of the main problems with cyberchondria is the biased way people are searching for and getting exposed to information. They are rarely searching in ways that will give them both sides of the story.

They are generally searching with biased questions—e.g., "are my symptoms cancer?"—and are paying more attention/clicking more on links that will be more likely to provide alarming information. They often look at nonscientific websites such as forums, social media, or fringe theories, which can emphasize a narrow focus on the possible, but improbable. Therefore, if you decide to use the internet for exposures, it is very important to be clear with yourself ahead of time about what content you are going to view, and for how long. How much information is enough?

We generally discourage patients from looking up what particular symptoms may mean. However, we often suggest patients do things like watch videos about others receiving medical news such as cancer diagnoses (such as for someone who has difficulty tolerating the uncertainty related to medical testing or receiving medical news). These exposures can also be quite helpful in getting a sense of what this experience looks like in real life, and how actual people process it and continue to live despite devastating news or difficult medical treatments. As we have mentioned many times above, when individuals are anxious, they are often overestimating how bad scary outcomes will be. Watching others go through difficult medical processes may disconfirm some overly negative beliefs about how awful the process is. In addition, we have often found that people have had several misconceptions about medical treatments, in terms of how risky, painful, or life-interfering they are. Watching the actual point-of-view testimony of people who have been through the experience or reading about the actual treatment online (ensuring that you do so with a reputable website!) can provide some corrective information about what the diagnosis or treatment process entails.

Should I Tell My Doctor I Am Anxious about Health?

Clinicians may vary on whether they think you should tell your physicians about your health anxiety. Often, therapists or patients fear that once a patient is labeled as "health-anxious," the medical provider may be more inclined to bias towards mental health explanations for symptoms, and inadvertently be dismissive of real issues.

Our view on this is that it is a personal choice, and you should weigh what you think is best for you given the nature of your illness anxiety. In our practice, we routinely encourage patients to inform their doctors about their health anxiety, with few exceptions. There are several reasons for this. One reason is that patients almost always report that their doctors are already quite aware they are anxious about health. Therefore, having the doctor aware that you have health anxiety can actually help them take more time to explain issues and recommendations to you appropriately, rather than being dismissive and assuming that you are just being dramatic or crying wolf. When medical providers are aware of mental health concerns, they may be in a better position to able to recommend, refer, or assess for psychiatry evaluations and medications when appropriate. In general, we have found that they have not been dismissive of patient's requests and inquiries when they are aware of illness anxiety, but typically more attentive, patient in explaining medical issues, coordinating care more when multiple providers are present, and more judicious about the tests they use. In turn, your doctor feels not left out of the loop, and now understands why you might show some anxious behaviors. They can become an integral part of your plan of tapering off excessive health behaviors. If you frequently visit doctors or have several medical providers, we highly suggest that you sign medical information-sharing consent forms with all of them so that they can all coordinate care to minimize unnecessary and repeated testing and visits. You may also want to limit care such that your general practitioner (primary care provider) is the "gatekeeper"—meaning that all referrals to specialists are on their recommendation and you do not seek out specialty care on your own. This can prevent you from getting too many cooks in the kitchen—so many medical providers involved that they are providing overlapping, confusing care.

6

Common Cognitive Distortions

Exposure Check-in and Troubleshooting

First, let's check in on how you have been doing with your initial exposures: did you do the exposure exercise you set out to do at the end of Chapter 5? Have you repeated it several times if possible? If not, can you do it now?

We recommend refraining from continuing in this workbook until you have practiced your first exposure several times, ideally for a prolonged period, and found that you have done it enough that your anxiety has noticeable reduced. Exposures are the most important part of treatment, and unfortunately, without doing them daily or near-daily, it is unlikely your symptoms will improve noticeably.

If you were able to practice the exposures, did it get any easier with time? Your anxiety is unlikely to be entirely gone, but you should notice it being easier than when you started! If it has gotten only slightly easier, you may simply need more time to practice. Stop here and take some time to really practice the exposure before moving on, in as many situations and as many times as possible. If you didn't see your anxiety reduce at all, or didn't complete the exposures, see below for a discussion of troubleshooting common issues.

DOI: 10.4324/9781032711355-6

Common Reasons for Not Doing Exposures

"I Didn't Get Time!"

One of the most common reasons we hear for not doing the exposures is "I was too busy—I didn't get time!" Unfortunately, effective exposure exercises do require quite a bit of time and effort. Take a moment to think about whether you are willing to devote at least 30 minutes a day to overcoming your anxiety. Certainly, you may be able to benefit from working on the skills at a slower pace, but for most people, to outweigh the anxious behaviors they are doing, dedication to daily practice is usually necessary. If you are already saying "no," the time commitment is more than I can handle, you may want to wait until you have more time to devote, so that you do not become discouraged. However, if lack of time is truly the problem, some people also get quite creative—we've seen people integrate exposures into eating meals, waiting in line, or while on mass transit to work!

If you are truly motivated to improve your anxiety and simultaneously very busy, you may also want to schedule time for you to do exposures for at least 30 minutes each day. We have had people enter this as an appointment in their planner/calendar, just as they would any other medical appointment they have to attend. Doing exposures regularly is an important part of the program, as procrastination tends to make anxiety worse in the long run. Think about being at a party, and you see someone across the room and you feel anxious and weird inside and want to avoid them at all costs. What would make your anxiety worse: going over and saying hello and getting it over with, or dodging them for hours at the party and always looking to see where they are? Right now, you have been taking the latter option. When we just confront our anxiety, it tends to go away a lot quicker compared to finding ways to avoid and dodge it.

"I Didn't Run into the Trigger This Week!"

Often people say that they did not do the exposure exercise as they were not confronted by the trigger over the course of the week. It is true that some exposure exercises do require us to wait for opportunities, such as a person who is afraid of getting their mammogram—we may need to wait until they have these appointments to practice them—you would not book repeated mammograms just for the sake of exposure! Most exposures can be sought out or induced in some way, even if it is only a part of the feared situation. For example, the person mentioned previously who is afraid of mammograms could watch videos of them being administered, or do imaginary exposures to receiving a cancer diagnosis after the mammogram—or things like that, depending on what the feared outcome is. If you look away from random medical posts on social media or ads that pop up in your browser, do not wait for them to cross your timeline or pop up—seek them out! Search for them and confront them in a prolonged, systematic fashion.

"It Was Too Distressing!"

The SUDS ratings are imperfect, and sometimes we overshoot an exposure. When that happens, we get into the situation where we find that it is much more anxiety-inducing than we thought it would be. No worries—if this happens, we suggest that if the anxiety is not very extreme, you don't escape or avoid the situation, but practice tolerating as much of it as you can. Generally, escaping or avoiding when you are at peak distress will feel extremely relieving and will only reinforce to your brain that the situation is terrifying, intolerable, and that you need to avoid it to survive. When possible, reduce the exposure slightly, but remain in the situation until your anxiety reduces a bit. For example, a patient who avoids hospitals might have an exposure goal of walking through a hospital for 30 minutes. However, when they get there, they realize their fear level is a 90 instead of the 40 they were anticipating. They may then decide to sit in the lobby or just walk one floor for the 30 minutes, rather than leaving the hospital entirely. Then walking throughout the hospital can be scheduled for a different day after sitting in the lobby has been practiced until it is much easier.

If You Did the Exposure Exercise(s), but It is Not Getting Easier with Repeated Practice

First, are you doing the exposure frequently, for long enough durations, and in enough different situations? Exposures may not get much easier without repeated practice. It is important get a significant "dose" of the anxiety trigger so that your brain learns that it can survive it, that feared outcomes are overestimated, and doesn't think that it was just some lucky fluke. The repeated exposure is more convincing to your brain than a one-off. In addition, we suggest, when possible, doing exposures in as many similar situations or ways as you can, to promote generalization. If people do an exposure with us only in-session, for example, they may feel that it gets easier, but only when they are in the safety of the clinic office. Or if they are practicing something like touching "germy" items in stores and do it only in one store, they are more likely to have it get easier in just that one store and still avoid and be uncomfortable in others. Therefore, we suggest that people do exposures in a variety of settings and ways.

Another thing to think about if you find that your exposures are not getting easier with repeated practice is whether you are truly confronting your feared outcomes. Sometimes people are missing the mark and confronting a health-related situation, but not really facing whatever it is about the situation that is the highest level of scary/fearful for them. As mentioned above, exposures tend to work best if you are really testing whether your anxious predictions are true or not. It is not unusual for exposures to remain somewhat anxiety-inducing until people really do face feared outcomes. Keep in mind that you may also gradually be decreasing safety behaviors, and will likely not experience maximum relief until all safety behaviors are suspended. For example, someone may want to reduce their excessive health-related reassurance-seeking, but may not feel that they can go cold turkey right away. Therefore, they may design several steps to reduce this safety behavior in increments, such as starting with a week of asking one reassurance question a day, then once a week the next week, then none the following week. Most people report that even the steps get easier with practice, but the real benefit comes from the last step: learning that you can tolerate life without any reassurance from family and friends that your signs and symptoms are not serious.

Setting This Week's Exposure

If you did your exposure and it reduced in anxiety, time to move onto the next one! Generally, in formal treatment we move on to the next exposure when a patient has practiced an exposure until it is around a 30 on the SUDS scale or lower. Write your next highest selected exposure on the Exposure Tracking Form below, and take a moment to note down in advance what you think your predictions are in terms of feared outcomes and anxiety level. We encourage you to start your exposure right now, or at the very least, if you are unable to start it now, schedule a time to do so, and one in which you are or someone else is holding you accountable. If you are feeling ambitious, you can do more than one exposure per week. Generally, we suggest that people work on one to three exposures per week; any more than that, and it can start to get overwhelming.

My Exposure Tracking Form

This week's exposure(s):

Anticipated discomfort (SUDS)	My anxious predictions: What do I think will happen when I do this (e.g., will I get hurt, ill, or die)? How uncomfortable will I be, and for how long?	Actual SUDS the final time I did the task this week	Actual outcome

Common Cognitive Distortions That Contribute to Anxiety

In Chapter 4, we discussed some thinking myths that are common in illness anxiety. Now that you have started doing exposures, you may notice more negative thinking patterns popping up. Have you had any anxious thoughts while doing or anticipating the exposures so far? What were they? If the initial exposures were fairly easy for you, are you having any anticipatory worries about future exposures? Write any anxious thoughts you can identify below.

_____

_____

_____

_____

While you are beginning your exposure plan, we'd like to further discuss some thinking problems that can maintain health anxiety and anxiety in general. Identifying and challenging these types of thinking has been part of cognitive behavioral therapy for decades, and can help you make the most of exposures.

Because you have strong thinking biases when you are anxious, stepping back and taking a closer look at your thoughts is important. To counter thinking biases, we encourage you to practice thinking like a scientist—that is, looking at all the information before making a conclusion. We don't want you to think overly positively, either—such as "Everything is fine, I will never get a serious medical condition!"—we view that as not very adaptive as well! Obviously, there is no way to be sure of an outcome such as that, and such a conclusion is just as distorted as anxious predictions that you surely will develop a serious medical condition. When people are anxious, they often base their conclusions on strong feelings, but feelings are not necessarily truth! You might be able to think of some occasions in your past in which you *felt* something was strongly accurate, but when you got more information, you discovered you were incorrect and it changed how you felt about the situation. We want you to factor in your emotions, but also practice systematically looking at the facts. We call this "thought challenging"—stepping back and weighing the evidence. Looking at the evidence and practicing thinking in new ways can reduce your health anxiety levels.[1]

Below is a list of common cognitive distortions that are often present in people who have anxiety or depression. CBT therapists often call these "distortions," because they are inaccurate, at least in part, but have been shown to fuel anxiety. They are interpretations we make in the moment that can happen quite reflexively, but that tend to be exaggerated and lead us to feeling worse. By identifying them and practicing correcting them so that they are accurate, we can reduce some anxiety.

You will notice that a lot of them have overlaps with the myths mentioned above, and with each other. We care less that you remember the names of the types of distortions (and as they have been used for many years, they may be called different things in different places). We rather hope that you will eventually able to understand what these thinking types are and begin to identify when they are present in your own thought patterns.

Review the list below carefully and try to think of examples of times when you have engaged in each of these thinking patterns. You will likely notice that sometimes you engage in these thinking patterns in areas other than illness anxiety as well, as most people engage in them from time to time (even the writers of this book!). Although you may find that not all of them apply to you, most people have engaged in most or all of them at times!

Common Cognitive Distortions in Health Anxiety

Magnification

Magnification is essentially "making a mountain out of a molehill." It is a form of catastrophizing, and is sometimes also called "overgeneralization." Magnification is when we take something that may be minor in and of itself, and focus on it intensively to the exclusion of other evidence, and make many more conclusions from it than are warranted. Another sign that this distortion may be present is exaggerated words like always, forever, never, everybody, nobody, and so on. Any time you begin a phrase or sentence with the words "What if …," that is also a sign you likely are catastrophizing. Few things in life are extreme and certain enough for these words to be accurate. Some examples of magnification distortions are listed below.

• "Doctors are always just looking to prescribe pills and make money; they don't care."	*These thoughts contain words like "always" and "anyone." These statements are unlikely to be literally true, and such blanket statements make it seem like things are bleaker than they are.*
• "If the doctor tells me I have diabetes, my life is over."	*Concluding that one's" life is over" because of a diagnosis of diabetes is extreme. While most people would consider this to be negative news, medical issues such as diabetes are generally considered to be very controllable and tolerable with treatment.*

Mind Reading

Mind reading occurs when we make assumptions about what others are thinking without sufficient evidence to jump to that conclusion. Most people think they are very good readers of what others are thinking, and frequently make very confident conclusions about what others must be thinking or feeling. However, these conclusions are debatable, and no one is a master at reading others—if they were, the FBI would hire them immediately for their special abilities! Instead, we make assumptions that are often based on ambiguous information, such as frowns, vague comments, or glances. Simultaneously, we tend to downplay or ignore other possible reasons for those behaviors (such as the other person being in a bad mood, feeling ill, being distracted or irritable about personal issues, and so on).

• "Anyone who noticed this mole would also be worried that it is skin cancer."	*These are assumptions about what others are thinking or feeling without conclusive evidence to prove that it was the case.*
• "The doctor didn't even seem to listen to me. He didn't care what I thought."	*These claims would be difficult to prove in court as they are based on your strong feelings, not facts.*

Fortune Telling

Fortune telling is another name for catastrophizing; it means that we are making predictions about what will happen, often without sufficient evidence that this is the case. Of course, these questionable predictions are always in the negative direction—no one is making predictions that they will win the lottery! Making these forecasts leaves us always prepared for the worst, feeling vigilant and apprehensive.

- "This arm pain is a sign I am having a heart attack!"

  This is a classic example of catastrophizing in illness anxiety—assuming that symptoms are signs of something serious. While serious illness may be possible, we ignore that there are many more likely outcomes that would explain the symptoms.

- "If I don't research about my health, I will miss something important to ask the doctor about, which will lead to them missing something crucial, which I will die from because I didn't catch it early enough."

  In addition to assuming the worst when we notice a symptom, and we might imagine a cascade of terrible events occurring. While this terrible chain of events might be possible, it is generally not what is probable based on the facts.

While we have discussed catastrophizing/fortune telling in chapter 2, it bears repeating here as it is the most common thinking distortion in illness anxiety. Take a moment now to look back on your cognitive monitoring forms that you have been doing so far. Specifically, look back on the predictions you made when you were feeling anxious—what did you think would happen? How often were you correct in your predictions? Most people recognize that they were almost never correct in what they thought would happen: that symptom was not a sign of something serious, the doctor didn't give them catastrophic news, they handled the situation better than they thought, and so on. What does tell you about how accurately you are thinking when you are anxious? It is important to practice taking your anxious predictions with a grain of salt. Alternatively, you can continue to let them bully you around into a life of fear over outcomes that do not occur as anticipated.

Labeling

Labeling is essentially name-calling. It occurs when we use derogatory labels that are excessive in their implication, and that do not reflect reality. Common labels are "idiot," "stupid," "selfish," "weak," "failure," "lazy," and so on. The problem with these labels is that no one is entirely stupid, weak, or selfish. These labels obscure nuances, and again make things seem bleaker than they are. In reality, there are gray areas. For example, we generally believe that people are not *lazy*, but rather they have varying motivations and abilities to do things based on a variety of factors such as physical energy, motivation, amount of reinforcement from the task, and their personal values and goals. This is a more nuanced and accurate way of describing behavior than a broad label such as "lazy."

- "People with chronic illnesses or disability are weak and a burden to others." — *This is a broad overgeneralization of an entire category of people. Certainly, there are many people who have chronic illness or injury who function excellently and excel in society.*

- "Doctors and healthcare systems are selfish and money-grubbing; they don't care what happens to me." — *This is a broad overstatement of the medical profession that cannot be entirely accurate. We agree that healthcare generally follows a business model in America and like any profession may have some limitations, and in rare cases healthcare professionals even engage in criminal actions to overbill or otherwise dupe or take advantage. However, this does not mean that all doctors act this way, and that doctors in general do not care about their patients.*

Emotional Reasoning

Emotional reasoning is when we make conclusions based on emotions, typically because we are feeling something so strongly. You may experience not feeling well, and then reason that you must be unwell because you feel unwell. You may not be able to pinpoint the exact feeling of being unwell, you just believe you are, therefore that equates to something being wrong with you. This reverse logic leads us to overfocus on our discomfort and excessively try to find causes of our anxiety.

In these cases of emotional reasoning, we start to base our conclusions and behaviors on scary outcomes that are possible, but not probable based on the evidence. Remember that when you are anxious, things often feel more dangerous or awful than they actually are or will be. Therefore, it's important to practice basing behavior on what is probable, not possible, just as you likely do in most other areas of your life! If you always based your actions on what is possible, you might never drive, socialize, leave your home, or do anything at all, because you might get in an accident, get attacked, rebuffed by others, or something else. However, if you are like most people, you do leave your home, drive, and/or interact with others, despite the risks. There are risks in everything you do. However, you do these things because they are important to you, so you accept the risks, and take appropriate precautions such as wearing a seat belt.

• "Because I feel so anxious that it might be a heart attack, I should just go to the ER again to get it ruled out."	*Both thoughts are conclusions and behaviors based on feelings, not evidence. It's important to recognize that while feelings can be strong, they may not reflect reality or signal that something is wrong.*
• "I know it's unlikely, but it feels like it could happen."	

"Should" Statements

"Should" statements are rules or expectations we have of how we think things "should" be, or what we think we or others "should" be doing. They are rules for living that we adopt from early caregivers or create in our own minds, and that may not be followed or agreed with by others. "Should" statements often are easy to identify as they often contain the words "should" or "should not."

However, sometimes they are more subtle, implied expectations. Some examples of "should" statements are as follows.

- "If it can be prevented, I should do all that I can to try and prevent it."

- "I shouldn't be this anxious all the time over these routine symptoms."

In the first two statements, the word "should" is clearly present. These are self-set rules that may or may not be helpful or correct.

- "I can't trust doctors; they didn't notice my signs and symptoms five years ago before I was diagnosed with cancer."

This is an example of a less obvious should statement. While there is not literally the phrase "should" or "shouldn't" in this thought, the implication of a should rule is there. For example, the statement implies that the doctor should have been able to detect the symptoms, and that one should not trust doctors if they appear to make mistakes or do not do what we expect.

Sometimes it is hard for people to understand why "should" statements might be problematic. We hear people say things like, "Well, isn't it good to have relatively high standards and aspire to be as healthy (or perfect) as possible?" So why might "should" statements be bad?

We find that "should" statements are often somewhat arbitrary—they are often rules we create from our own rule book. The problem with this is that no one else is reading or following our rule book! Then we get upset when others do not respect our rules. In addition, we often get upset with ourselves. Because the rules are often somewhat arbitrary, they are often too high for us to meet. People often set "should" rules that are just out of reach, making it feel demoralizing when they (or others) fall short of them again and again. Rather than update their rules, they usually replace them with more "shoulds": "I shouldn't feel this bad" or "I should try harder next time," etc., leading to a cycle of negativity, typically without getting closer to goals over time, and never feeling like they are doing quite well enough.

We also commonly hear "I should not feel this way" or "I should feel the way I felt before all this anxiety happened to me."

Can you set goals for yourself that do not lead you to feel awful from the statement itself? We can immediately feel like we have failed ourselves when we phrase statements in this manner. Can you replace these words with something like, "I'd like to start …"? Compassion with yourself is the name of the game here.

Practicing Talking Back to Your Anxious Thoughts

Do you see any of the cognitive distortion thinking patterns (magnification, mind reading, fortune telling, labeling, emotional reasoning, "should" statements) in your self-monitoring from the past week or the anxious thoughts you listed earlier? We encourage you to get very familiar with all these types of thinking so that you can identify them.

Given that anxious thoughts can be quite distorted and greatly impact how we feel, it is important to not only recognize that there is distorted thinking present, but then to begin to work on changing it. Simply being aware of the distortions is helpful, but the real improvements tend to follow systematic and repeated practice in challenging, or talking back to, these thoughts by correcting them when they may not be accurate.

We do this by having you write out your anxious thoughts and formally begin to develop corrections to those thoughts, in which you re-write the thought without the distortions present, making sure the thoughts are factual and correct, rather than exaggerated.

On the table below called "Thought Challenging Form" you will see a form for practicing this. On below we also include an example form to give you a sense of what it might look like. You may want to make copies or use additional sheets of paper if you have more entries, as the more you practice this, the better! Take out the form and challenge your thoughts when you notice an upswing in anxiety.

The Thought-challenging Form looks a lot like the form you completed to monitor your thoughts, but has one additional column that is very important: a column to write a corrected version of your thoughts. So you will first write your anxious thoughts in the second column, and in the third column re-write your thoughts without distortions. The corrected thoughts should be literally accurate thoughts that look at the evidence that is available to you, taking a hard and careful look at all the evidence, not just the evidence that is consistent with your fears. What does the evidence really say about this situation? Do you have enough evidence to make a conclusion? What might you argue if you were a lawyer for the other side of the argument?

First, a couple tips for practicing this thought-challenging. One problem people run into is that they notice themselves thinking in questions, which can be hard to challenge. Usually, but not always, these are "What if …?" types of questions, such as ""What if my cancer comes back?" or "Could be it be a sign of a stroke?" To make these easier to challenge, we typically change these to statements, to reflect the prediction you are implying to yourself. Therefore, "What if my cancer comes back?" might become "My cancer will come back, and I won't be able to handle it," or "Could it be a stroke?" might change to "My headache could be a sign of stroke, and I can't tolerate the uncertainty of not checking in with my doctor." Also distinguish between what you are thinking and what you are feeling—they are often very different! If you feel an emotion, ask yourself what interpretation you were making that might have contributed to that emotion. For example, a statement of "I feel sad" is identifying an emotion. When we ask "Why might you feel sad?", the patient may say something like, "I did not like how the day went. It was unpredictable and a mess. I couldn't refrain from checking my weight." See the difference? The latter is the thought, or interpretation, that we are interested in taking a closer look at.

Second, sometimes people report somewhat of a disconnect between what they feel and what they *believe* on paper. For now, that discrepancy is expected and OK. It often takes quite a bit of challenging practice for feelings to "catch up" with what you believe according to the evidence. For now, it's most important that your corrected thoughts are thoughts that you believe as fact—that you can say you believe, despite what you feel. In doing so, you may find that you believe that some of your anxious thoughts are true. However, most people discover that at least some of their anxious thoughts are exaggerated or inaccurate, at least in part. In considering whether your cognitive challenges are true and accurate, consider whether they are based in fact. A way of thinking about this is to use the "court" test—would this statement fly in a court of law, or would a judge say that there is not enough evidence to convict? There is a reason why feelings are not allowed as evidence in court—feelings are often incorrect! We may *feel* someone is guilty of a crime, but that does not mean they are. Rather, we look at the evidence to make our conclusions.

Finally, it's OK if you find yourself challenging similar themes—it's not unusual for the same types of thoughts to keep coming up! Sometimes patients come in with only one or two entries, and we express surprise that they only felt anxious once over the past week! They then note that they felt anxious nearly daily, but did not challenge the thoughts each time because the thoughts were always the same. If this happens, practice challenging them every time. Thoughts that keep recurring are usually the most important thought patterns to challenge. However, make sure you are challenging the thoughts that are truly bothersome. In doing so, you should notice at least some slight improvement in anxiety. If not, continue to ask yourself what other implications or assumptions you may have about the situation that warrant additional challenging. Use the Thought-challenging Form as a tool in the moment to help your anxious thinking. It will not make anxiety go away, but if you are doing it correctly, it should shave a couple degrees of distress off your anxious thinking.

Thought-challenging Form (Example)

Trigger (What started the anxiety? Or what was going on at the time when you noticed your anxiety spike?)	Thoughts (Also, if that thought were true, what would be so bad about that to you?)	What distortions are present? What are the facts? Re-write your thoughts without distortions.
I woke up after another night of poor sleep after several nights in a row.	I remember reading somewhere that lack of sleep is related to lowered immune function for people my age. This is going to make it more likely I get severely ill and end up in the hospital, where I will be likely to catch even more illnesses.	I don't have a <u>chronic</u> lack of sleep, it is intermittent. This is also fortune telling: it may impact immune function, but I have no signs of that. I don't know for sure it will lead to severe illness; I can't predict the future. Most people go to the hospital to get better, and I know the hospitals are cautious about trying to prevent contagions, that's their job.
I noticed a small rash-like mark on my neck.	I haven't seen anything like this before. I should call the doctor. It might be something serious, and if I don't catch it early, it could become a real issue.	This might be magnification. I have been tempted to call the doctor many times before and the visit hasn't been that informative; they couldn't find anything wrong with me. I don't have any proof it's something serious; in fact, I nearly always think it's serious and it never is.
My doctor didn't respond to my emails asking questions about the results of my biopsy. The nurse said I had to schedule an appointment to ask the questions.	Doctors should respond to people who are anxious about their test results. I should change doctors to get someone more responsive.	This is a "should" statement. It's possible my doctor is somewhat frustrated with me because I email her after nearly every test with many questions, which is time-consuming for her. She has contacted me in the past if there was reason to be concerned about the results.

Thought-challenging Form

Trigger (What started the anxiety? Or what was going on at the time when you noticed your anxiety spike?)	Thoughts (Also, if that thought were true, what would be so bad about that to you?)	What distortions are present? What are the facts? Re-write your thoughts without distortions.

7

Interoceptive Exposures

Check-in on Treatment Homework

Thought-challenging Practice

First, let's check in on the thought-challenging practice. Have you been practicing completing the Thought-challenging Form in Chapter 6 over the past week? This generally works best if you use it as a tool in the moment to help you feel better. If possible, try to remember to take it out and work through your thoughts each time you notice a substantial upswing in feeling anxious about health.

When it works correctly, the thought-challenging should reduce your distress about the situation by at least a few degrees. It will not remove the distress entirely or take the problem away, of course, but it should bring your discomfort down a notch or two when you practice thinking realistically about the situation. If you are finding that you are still highly distressed after you do the challenging, we encourage you to continue to ask yourself what interpretations you are making that are truly bothering you.

DOI: 10.4324/9781032711355-7

Taking a look at your Thought-challenging Form, what are the most common cognitive distortions that you find yourself engaging in? For example, do you notice high rates of fortune telling (thinking the worst)? Or do you notice patterns like lots of "should" statements, feeling that you need to figure out symptoms *right now*, or chronic mistrust of doctors? Being aware of the reflexive thinking patterns that you tend to engage in is truly important to be able to step back from them and evaluate whether they are something you truly believe and want to base your behavior on. We often think that we are more aware of these cognitive interpretations than we actually are. Don't skimp on the thought-challenging!

We encourage you to keep up with the thought-challenging for at least a few weeks (some people decide to do it for much longer, as the more practice, the better!). Therefore, we have included another Thoughtchallenging Form below so that you can continue your efforts.

Thought-challenging Form

Trigger (What started the anxiety? Or, what was going on at the time when you noticed your anxiety spike?)	Thoughts (Also, if that thought were true, what would be so bad about that, to you?)	What distortions are present? What are the facts? Re-write your thoughts without distortions.

Exposure Practice

Let's also check back in on how you have been doing with your exposures: did you do the exposure exercise you set out to do this week? Have you repeated it several times if possible? If not, can you do it now?

If you did your exposure, what did you learn about your predictions versus the actual outcome? Did you write this down on the Exposure Tracking Form? If not, do it now. Were your predictions correct, in terms of what feared outcomes you were telling yourself would happen, and how anxious you thought you would be and for how long? If your feared outcomes did happen, how did you handle them? Was it better or worse than you thought it would be? Essentially, what did you learn from this experiment? Do you have enough evidence to make you feel relatively sure in your conclusions, or do you need more data?

Once you have practiced your exposure exercise for at least a week and the anxiety has reduced, you can move on to the next item in your hierarchy. There is another Exposure Form below below for you to write down the specific exposure(s) you plan to do this week and to track your predictions about what will happen.

This week's exposure(s):

Anticipated discomfort (SUDS)	My anxious predictions: What do I think will happen when I do this (e.g., will I get hurt, ill, or die)? How uncomfortable will I be, and for how long?	Actual SUDS the final time I did the task this week	Actual outcome

Interoceptive Exposures

So far, you have been practicing doing exposures to confront your health anxiety cues and reduce safety behaviors. In addition to doing these exposures, we suggest doing another type of exposure called *interoceptive* exposure. The word "interoceptive" refers to internal experiences, or bodily sensations. This means the focus of the exposures is on the experience of anxiety in the body, or somatic sensations.

The bodily sensations associated with anxiety are highly individualized, and different people experience different physical sensations. In addition, the physical sensations, signs, and symptoms that make them anxious about their health are not necessarily the same ones they have when they are strongly anxious. Figure 7.1 shows some sensations people might experience when they are feeling especially anxious, and are considered part of the body's anxiety response.

This list is not exhaustive, and you may experience many of the sensations in this list, only a few of them, or none. Are there

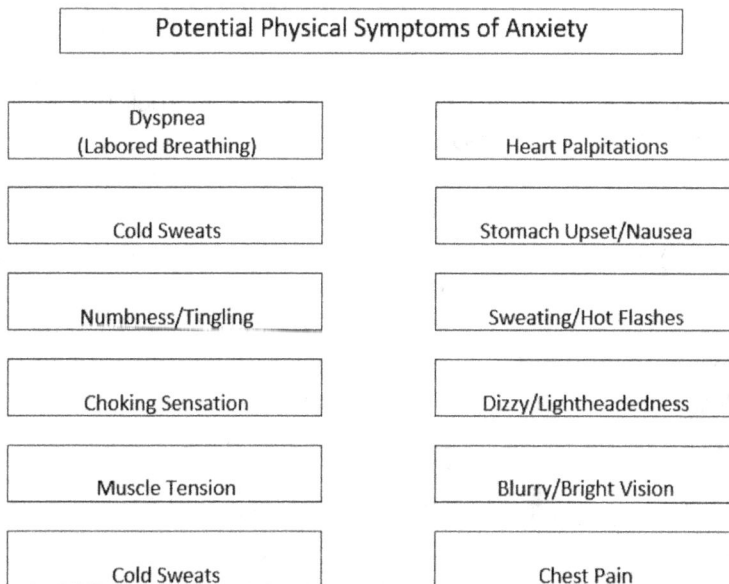

Potential Physical Symptoms of Anxiety	
Dyspnea (Labored Breathing)	Heart Palpitations
Cold Sweats	Stomach Upset/Nausea
Numbness/Tingling	Sweating/Hot Flashes
Choking Sensation	Dizzy/Lightheadedness
Muscle Tension	Blurry/Bright Vision
Cold Sweats	Chest Pain

FIGURE 7.1 Physical anxiety symptoms

any physical sensations you notice when you are anxious that are not listed in Figure 7.1?

As you know, individuals with health anxiety are often worried about physical signs and symptoms. However, as mentioned in Chapter 6 on thinking patterns, regular physical symptoms are common even in healthy individuals, and they are commonly experienced when people are anxious! However, people with illness anxiety are more likely to have a catastrophic sense of these physical sensations. Even if you do not experience any of the sensations in Figure 7.1 when you are anxious, because you have health anxiety you are likely to notice physical sensations and catastrophize about them. Therefore, an important component of exposure for illness anxiety is to do *internal* exposures (also known as interoceptive exposures). This involves repeatedly and intentionally inducing the physical sensations that are associated with anxiety. We do this for multiple reasons.

Getting Used to Physical Sensations
Because you are hypervigilant to and oversensitive to physical sensations, you likely try to avoid having them. You might be doing this without being aware of it. This may include avoiding some situations that trigger physical sensations, such as exercise, alcohol or caffeine use, or amusement park rides, and so on. However, because you are likely to try to not "rock the boat" with internal physical sensations, your body is less used to having them. Therefore, they are more likely to send up red flags to your brain when they occur. Therefore, by repeatedly experiencing them, your body can get more used to having them. This is like training for fighter pilots and individuals who work on boats—when they first start training, they may feel extremely sick and have a variety of physical sensations. However, with repeated practice and exposure to these situations, the body can calibrate a bit and these experiences become more tolerable.

Learning That You Can Tolerate Physical Sensations
Because you are likely avoiding physical sensations to some degree, you are not used to having them. Also, because you may

try to suppress or avoid them, you are less likely to learn that if you allow yourself to have them without doing anything to try to make them go away, they will pass with time, and that while unpleasant, they are tolerable. We can walk around with a pebble in our shoe, and yet we aren't fearful that it means our foot needs to be cut off. We can tolerate a certain level of discomfort.

Learning That Physical Sensations Do Not Lead to Medical Catastrophe (Testing Your Predictions)

Your body needs to learn the difference between experiencing a sensation as uncomfortable versus anxiety or fear-provoking. As described in Chapter 5 on exposure, one of the main reasons for doing exposures is to test your anxious fears, as when people are anxious, they tend to think in biased ways. When it comes to physical sensations, this means that people are often afraid that if they allow physical sensations to continue and do not try to figure them out, awful things will happen. For example, they may be thinking that they they if they do not try to do anything about the sensations, they will not detect a medical problem early enough for it to be treatable. Or they may worry that the sensations will worsen until they are painful. Or they may simply fear the experience of sitting with uncertainty. Exposing yourself to physical sensations can help you discover that if you do not do anything about your symptoms, catastrophic outcomes are unlikely to occur, and that if negative outcomes occur, you can handle them better than you thought! Also, you will practice the most important part: tolerating sitting with uncertainty.

Practicing Different Behaviors When Physical Sensations Arise

Part doing of the interoceptive exposures is to practice not feeding into the cycle of uncomfortable negative sensations. Often when people notice uncomfortable symptoms, their first reaction is to think, "Oh no!" They might reflexively tense up, fidget, and become vigilant to sensations, and notice that their heart rate has increased because now they are apprehensive, and the cycle of anxiety spins upward. Therefore, when practicing interoceptive exposures, we encourage you to bring on the sensation and practice calmly accepting the sensations, rather than tensing up and adding to the anxiety cycle. Allow the sensation to be while relaxing your muscles as much a possible.

Medical Readiness for Interoceptive Exposures

The interoceptive exposures that are listed in this book are designed to mimic sensations most people experience at times in ordinary life, and therefore are generally quite safe. They generally induce a level of physical sensations that can be mildly uncomfortable, but tolerable. We view them as quite similar, for the most part, to sensations that arise when you do mild to moderate exercise.

However, if you have a medical condition for which your doctor has directly instructed you to minimize certain activities, you may want to refrain from that interoceptive exposure. We obviously do not recommend doing interoceptive exposure that would be likely to exacerbate injury or medical issues. Occasionally, patients do have diagnosed medical issues (e.g., serious cardiological problems or pulmonary problems) that would be worsened by some of the interoceptive exposures, and in those cases we avoid them or obtain the doctor's approval to do them. However, we encourage you to exercise caution about getting medical approval, since this can be a safety behavior. In our treatment facilities, most people do all the below interoceptive exposures without consulting their doctor. Generally, what we tell patients is that if your doctor has not directly told you to avoid that type of activity, let's give it a go, and we can start at a somewhat lower level if possible (e.g., doing it for half the recommended time). Sometimes patients are avoiding exposures that would be beneficial because they are afraid of the sensations, or overestimating the impact they will have on their medical symptoms when this is not medically warranted, but rather part of the health anxiety. They may be looking for extra reassurance by having their doctor sign off on these exposures as "safe." Remember that the point of the interoceptive exposure is to bring on mildly uncomfortable physical sensations and to tolerate some uncertainty.

If you are unsure about whether your medical issues will be impacted, you may want to show your treating physician the list of interoceptive exposures to ensure that none of them are likely to worsen medical issues for you. Given that most patients we encounter are health-anxious, they have often been through sufficient medical evaluation and been informed by their doctors that there is no medical condition, or at least no condition that warrants the level of symptoms they are experiencing. However, if you avoid healthcare or have not been evaluated by a physician in several years and are experiencing symptoms, you may want have a physical with your provider to ensure you are in decent health prior to initiating the interoceptive exposures.

It is not uncommon for people to have some sensations linger for minutes to hours after the exposures (especially after doing several in a row). While the point of the interoceptive exposures is to induce and practice tolerating physical sensations, we encourage you to discontinue and first consult your doctor if you notice any negative lasting effects that you think may be related to the exposures. If you have medical conditions you think would be exacerbated by exposures, or are unsure, you may also want to consider doing them with a therapist who is trained in CBT or health psychology. For most individuals who are in reasonably good health, the interoceptive exposures should be bodily sensations your body is designed to have: somewhat uncomfortable, but tolerable!

Doing Interoceptive Exposures

Below you will find a list of some of the most common interoceptive exposures we practice with health-anxious patients in our clinic. Even if you find that you are only bothered by very specific types of medical symptoms (e.g., cardiac, respiratory, digestive), we usually encourage patients to go through the entire core list, doing each of the exposures a few times and rating the discomfort of each, as we have found that individuals with illness anxiety tend to be alarmed by a great variety of weird new physical sensations, so the more you practice, the better! As you go, use the Interoceptive Rating Form later in the chapter to rate each exposure on two dimensions: how much anxiety the sensations caused for you, and how strong the sensations were for you (i.e., just how strong the sensations were compared to how strongly you have ever had them, setting aside how anxious or distressing they were).

In the second column, take a moment to really pay attention to the sensations you have during the exposure, and practice sitting quietly for at least 30 seconds after the exposure to notice any new sensations you have while you are recovering. Often the sensations that people might have during the while doing the exposure (e.g., mild nausea while spinning) might be different from those that occur immediately when they stop (dizziness, shaky/blurry vision, "blood rushing to the head" feeling). It is important to note that while the descriptions of the interoceptive exposures note several example sensations, internal sensations may vary, which is why we ask you to record your personal experience. As usual, the first row on the form is an example entry to show you how the exposures might be recorded.

Core List of Interoceptive Exposures

Straw Breathing

Straw breathing is usually used to induce sensations of not being able to get a full breath. People doing this exposure often report sensations such as chest tightening, dry mouth, lightheadedness, jaw tightening or pressure, or chest pressure. To do this exposure, take a small coffee stirrer-size straw, plug your nose, and close your mouth around the straw. Take all breaths in and out *only* through the straw, ensuring that you are not otherwise breathing through your mouth or nose. Usually, we have people breathe in this way continuously as long as they can to start with, working their way up until they can do it for at least two minutes straight without breaks. Most people find this one of the more difficult exposures to do. In fact, most patients when they first try this exposure say that breathing for two minutes straight only through a small straw can't be done! However, at the end

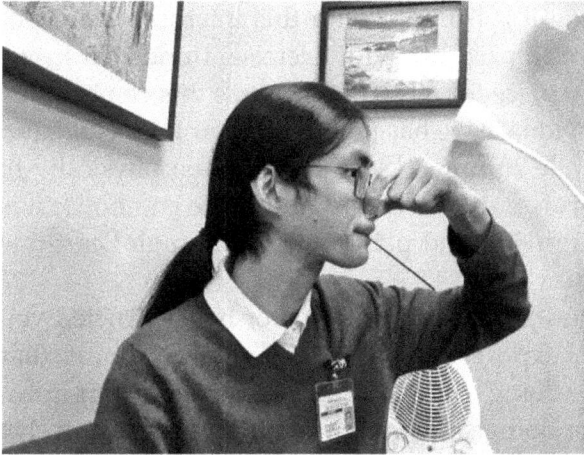

FIGURE 7.2 Straw breathing

of treatment after much practice, they have all been able to do it, some for much longer periods of time!

Small coffee stirrer straws are preferred and are available in most coffee shops or cafes, but if you absolutely do not have access to them, you may also use a normal straw or hollowed-out pen as a tube, but as this size tube allows for much more air, we usually encourage people do some exercise (e.g., 30 jumping jacks) immediately before breathing through the larger straw to better simulate the effect of constrained breathing.

Running in Place

This interoceptive exposure is designed to induce most of the physical sensations that occur when people do cardiovascular exercise, such as high heart rate, shortness of breath, and/or muscle weakness or strain. We typically have people run in place for a continuous 60 sessions, but depending on how physically fit you are, how much you exercise already and how mobile you are, other options include activities such as walking at a brisk pace up a flight of stairs or doing planks or squats. If you have medical conditions, you can also ask your doctor for advice on appropriate cardiovascular exercise (they are often happy that you are considering it!). The idea with this interoceptive exposure is to raise your heart rate with exercise. In our clinic, we have people run in place for 60 seconds, but as this can be quite easy for most individuals, we have them lift their knees high (up past the waist) while running. Most people (even physically fit ones!) find that this is quite strenuous, and at the end notice it is difficult to keep up with, and point out at least high heart rate and ragged breathing.

If you cannot run in place or your doctor has instructed you not to, replacement exposures that induce similar cardiovascular symptoms include doing a plank for one minute (on your arms, not your hands), or doing squats for two minutes consecutively.

Hyperventilation

Hyperventilation is a great interoceptive exposure to induce a variety of physical sensations, and tends to be one of the strongest ones for many people. To do hyperventilation, we suggest heavy, rapid breathing (like a dog panting) continuously for one minute. Make sure you are cycling air in and out fairly rapidly, and with a fair amount of pressure. Most people will report experiencing sensations like lightheadedness, chest pressure, dry mouth, bright or blurry vision, slight headache/head pressure, or dizziness.

Sweating/hot Flashes

Often when people are hypervigilant to physical sensations, they try to avoid situations that feel warm or stuffy. They might be doing things like making sure they always have layers of clothing on to remove as needed, water with them, or have a window cracked open when they are driving. There are many ways to induce warmth that can be appropriate for this exposure, such as wearing several layers of clothing, sitting near a heater, or sitting in your car with all the windows up and the heat on highest setting. Typically, you only need to do this for a few minutes, but we encourage you do it so that you at least notice some sweating and mild discomfort. Typically, people doing this exposure report sensations like feeling hot, sweaty, or mild nausea.

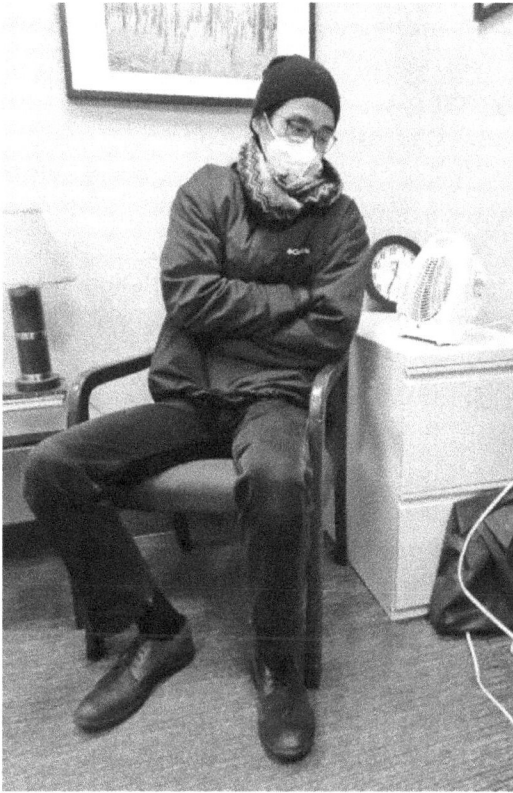

FIGURE 7.3 Body heat

Choking Feelings

There are several ways to mimic a feeling of throat tightening or choking. One of the best ways we have found to do this is called rapid swallowing. In rapid swallowing, you try to swallow as many times as you can as fast as you can for 30 seconds. Most people find that after a handful of swallows, their throat starts to tighten up and it becomes difficult to continue swallowing. Other options to practice having these types of sensations include eating crackers with no liquid, wearing a scarf tied around your neck snugly and swallowing, or breathing only with your mouth for a few minutes.

Chest/abdominal Pressure

There are several ways to induce chest or stomach pressure feelings. These include wearing an overly tight belly band or large belt to moderately compress breathing or add a feeling of tightness. Alternatively, you may lie on your back with a pile of books (usually 3–7 lbs.) on your chest or abdomen while you breathe in and out for a few minutes. See Figure 7.4 for a depiction of this interoceptive. A final way of doing this is chest stretching (see Figure 7.5): sit up straight in chair that has a back. Interlace your fingers behind your head. Next, tilt your head back as far as possible without moving your back or position. Finally, bring your elbows back as far as you can, as if you were trying to touch them behind your head, while keeping your fingers interlaced behind your head. Now, while in this position, take some deep chest breaths—the kind you would do at the doctor's office—for a minute or so. If you are doing the exposure correctly, you should notice that it is somewhat difficult to take deep breaths—your chest may feel strained, and breathing may be ragged.

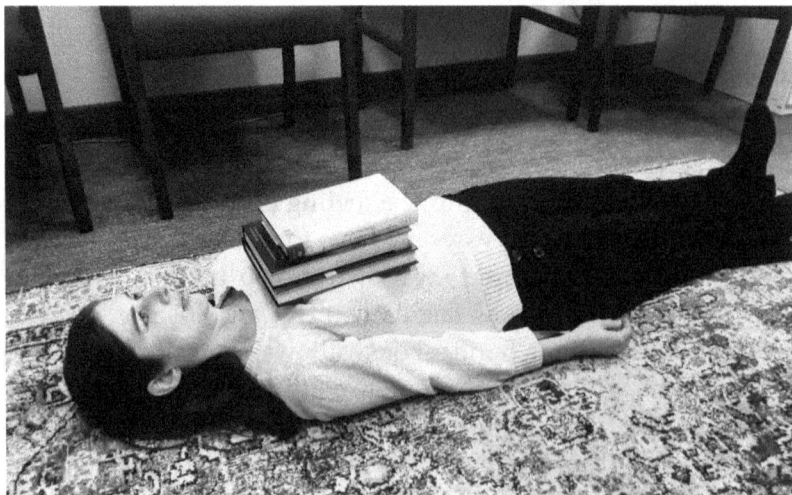

FIGURE 7.4 Chest pressure

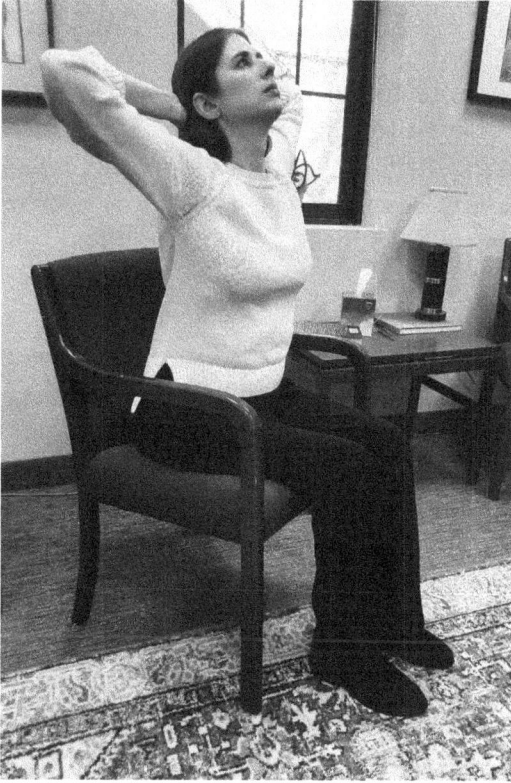

FIGURE 7.5 Chest stretching

Dizziness

Generally, the best way to induce feelings of dizziness is to spin around. You may do this standing, but if you have a swivel chair available, you can also spin in a chair. We suggest spinning at a moderate pace for at least 30 seconds. After doing this, most people will notice feelings of dizziness: mild nausea, lightheadedness, blurry or shaky vision, and so on. This is an important exposure to sit with for at least a minute after spinning, practicing noticing and tolerating physical sensations, as most people find that the strongest sensations with this exposure occur immediately after they stop spinning.

Head shaking or head rolling can other good, usually slightly less extreme ways to induce light dizziness. Head shaking involves rapidly moving your head from side to side, as if you were saying "no" vigorously for 30 seconds. To do head rolling, move your chin down to your chest, then roll it in a circle until your head is upright. Continue to move in circles at a moderate pace for 30 seconds. You may want to avoid this one if you have neck or back issues. Driving over hilly areas and winding roads, or riding amusement park rides can also be a great way to practice getting used to feelings of dizziness!

Lightheadedness

Another way to induce lightheadedness is to sit in a chair and bend over, putting your head upside down in between your legs. The more you can hold your head upside down, the better. Hold that position for 60 seconds, then fairly quickly shift back up to an upright sitting position. Most people doing this will notice a "rushing" feeling when they sit back up, possibly with some lightheadedness. They may also notice some different sensations when their head is upside down, such as the head feeling heavy (blood rushing to the head) or head pressure.

Eye Sensitivity

A common physical sensation related to anxiety that can make people anxious is bright or blurry vision. To induce this, we typically have patients stare directly into a flashlight for 30 seconds, and then look away and try to read some written material such as a book. Most patients report bright or spotty vision. An alternative is to look or walk around a bit wearing glasses with a prescription that slightly not a match for your own eyesight.

Muscle Tension

To do muscle tensing, sit in a chair. Then attempt to tense all your muscles at once, from head to toe, holding the tension for one full minute without breaks. Try to tense up your muscles so much that it is hard to do, but not so hard that you cramp up. Most people report that this position is hard to hold for a full minute, as it is like exercise. During the tensing, people often report muscle tightness, heart racing, and sometimes shaking. After the exercise, patients often report a sense of warmth or "rushing" feeling as they unclench and muscles go back to a relaxed state.

Numbness/tingling

Numbness or tingling can be hard to induce, but sometimes patients practice this by wearing tight fitting clothing. Another way to do this is to place a book or umbrella tight into in your armpit, then press your arm down for 30 seconds. Most people will notice a feeling of their arm "falling asleep"—usually marked by numbness in arm/fingers and tingling. This is an especially good exposure for individuals who are afraid of arm pain being a sign of cardiac issues despite a lack of substantial cardiac risk factors. You may also want to try tightly squeezing your hands or feet for three minutes. For many people, this will lead to extremities feeling numb and/or tingly.

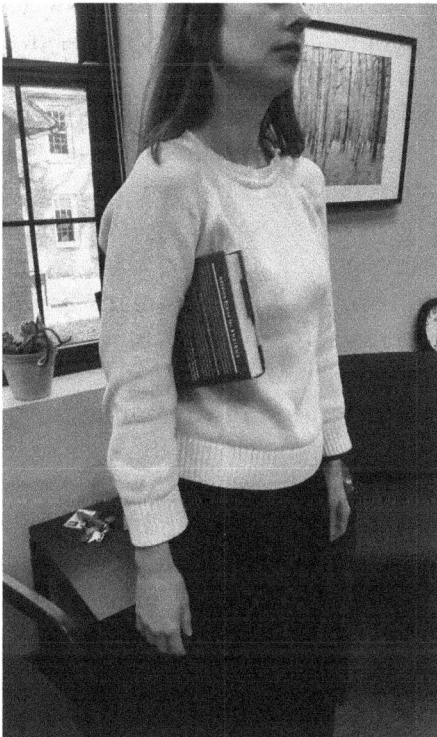

FIGURE 7.6 Arm numbness

Sour Stomach

Patients are often concerned about a variety of digestive symptoms. Therefore, we encourage a variety of exposures that target physical sensations related to eating: eating spicy food, eating food you have never tried before (or in a new restaurant/place if you are only eating at "safe" or familiar locations), taking longer breaks between eating, eating when you do not feel your best, or overeating for a meal to get a sensation of fullness. You can also push on your stomach uncomfortably for a period of one minute (where your esophagus meets your stomach, where it branches off at the bottom of your sternum).

Derealization/depersonalization

Derealization or depersonalization are the psychological names for feeling spacy, out-of-body, like things do not seem real, or seem dreamlike. This is one of the interoceptive sensations that can be the hardest to induce, as the subjective experience of it can be quite different for different people. One study[1] suggested that one of the most reliable ways to simulate this may be to sit in a dark room with a strobe light (obviously do not do this exposure if you have any history of photosensitive seizures). While you likely do not have access to a strobe light, you may be able to take advantage of opportunities to do so, such as party events, concerts, or haunted houses. Alternatively, a way to induce some derealization feelings can be spot staring. To do spot staring, pick a very tiny spot around three to five feet from you. Stare at that spot continuously for two minutes without looking away. Some people report a sensation of tunnel vision or dreamlike fuzziness. Some people have also done this by staring at themselves in a mirror, or staring at their hand, for two minutes while repeating their name or a phrase. While this may sound odd, some people have reported that they start to feel a funny sense—like when you say a word many times and it stops sounding like an actual word! Really, engaging in any visually deceiving exercise will result in a derealization/depersonalization experience. It is important to test many of the options listed above, as what works for one person will not work for another, and vice versa.

Interoceptive Rating Form

Interoceptive exposure	What physical sensations did you notice?		Rate strength of sensations (0–10)	Rate anxiety (0–10)
Example: Hyperventilation (60 seconds)	-ightheadedness, dry mouth, brief bright/ blurry vision, slightly nauseous, mild headache	Trial 1:	6	7
		Trial 2:	5	6
		Trial 3:	4	5
Straw breathing (2 minutes)		Trial 1:		
		Trial 2:		
		Trial 3:		
Running in place (bringing knees high, 60 seconds)		Trial 1:		
		Trial 2:		
		Trial 3:		
Hyperventilation (60 seconds)		Trial 1:		
		Trial 2:		
		Trial 3:		

Interoceptive exposure	What physical sensations did you notice?		Rate strength of sensations (0–10)	Rate anxiety (0–10)
Sweating/hot flashes		Trial 1:		
		Trial 2:		
		Trial 3:		
Choking feelings (rapid swallowing, 30 seconds)		Trial 1:		
		Trial 2:		
		Trial 3:		
Chest/abdominal pressure		Trial 1:		
		Trial 2:		
		Trial 3:		
Dizziness (spinning, 30 seconds)		Trial 1:		
		Trial 2:		
		Trial 3:		
Lightheadedness		Trial 1:		
		Trial 2:		
		Trial 3:		

Interoceptive exposure	What physical sensations did you notice?		Rate strength of sensations (0–10)	Rate anxiety (0–10)
Eye sensitivity		Trial 1:		
		Trial 2:		
		Trial 3:		
Muscle tension (60 seconds)		Trial 1:		
		Trial 2:		
		Trial 3:		
Sour stomach		Trial 1:		
		Trial 2:		
		Trial 3:		
Numbness/ Tingling		Trial 1:		
		Trial 2:		
		Trial 3:		
Derealization/ Depersonalization		Trial 1:		
		Trial 2:		
		Trial 3:		

The point of the exposures is to induce normal and mildly to moderately uncomfortable bodily sensations, and practice tolerating them. We have found that in the clinic, sometimes people end exposures prematurely or only do them half-heartedly, so they do not induce many physical sensations. If your ratings of physical sensations and anxiety were both low (i.e., all under 5), we encourage you to go back and try to persist with practicing the exposures for slightly longer periods to see if they can induce stronger sensations, and to ensure that you are doing the exposure fully without protective behaviors. For example, if you found that running in place for one minute was too easy (this is rare!), you may want to try running in place for 90 seconds while bringing your knees slightly higher. It can also be helpful to do several of the interoceptive exposures in a row, as this can lead to a build-up of several bodily sensations. You can also combine more than one interoceptive exposure to create a harder overall exposure and really challenge and improve your ability to tolerate levels of distress, such as by hyperventilating in a warm room, or running in place and then spinning. Again, use your judgment to ensure you are not worsening any medical conditions if you have any, but most of the exposures described are considered relatively routine and safe, and are designed to mimic normal bodily sensations people might encounter.

Once you have tried all the exposures in the core list at least three times, we suggest you select your top three interoceptive exposures that lead to the strongest sensations and most distress for you. Once you have selected your top three, practice those interoceptive exposures at least three times as day for at least three weeks. After three weeks, you can start to get creative and combine different interoceptive exposures to make them more difficult. For example, you can breathe through a straw and do a plank at the same time. Ensure while you are doing the exposures that you stay focused on the feelings you are experiencing. You can also increase the complexity of the exposure by combining it with intentionally thinking about your fears. For example, you could repetitively say to yourself "I want to experience a heart attack and be disabled" while also performing a one-minute plank and breathing through a straw. This may sound like a very challenging exposure, but the more you confront your anxiety, the less your mind and body will be afraid of it going forward. We will discuss more on imaginal/verbal exposures in the next chapter as well.

Below we include a template form for tracking your exposure practice across the week. We suggest you practice your top three interoceptive exposures daily for at least a few weeks. You can also practice more than your top three if there were many that bothered you. You may want to continue to practice them, especially the ones with sensations that bother you, if you feel anxious about them in the future.

My Interoceptive Exposure Practice Tracking Form

My top 3 interoceptive exposures	Monday	Tuesday	Wednesday	Thursday	Friday	Saturday	Sunday
1)	Trial 1:	Trial 1:	Trial 1:	Trial 1:	Trial 1:	Trial 1:	Trial 1:
	Trial 2:	Trial 2:	Trial 2:	Trial 2:	Trial 2:	Trial 2:	Trial 2:
	Trial 3:	Trial 3:	Trial 3:	Trial 3:	Trial 3:	Trial 3:	Trial 3:
2)	Trial 1:	Trial 1:	Trial 1:	Trial 1:	Trial 1:	Trial 1:	Trial 1:
	Trial 2:	Trial 2:	Trial 2:	Trial 2:	Trial 2:	Trial 2:	Trial 2:
	Trial 3:	Trial 3:	Trial 3:	Trial 3:	Trial 3:	Trial 3:	Trial 3:
3)	Trial 1:	Trial 1:	Trial 1:	Trial 1:	Trial 1:	Trial 1:	Trial 1:
	Trial 2:	Trial 2:	Trial 2:	Trial 2:	Trial 2:	Trial 2:	Trial 2:
	Trial 3:	Trial 3:	Trial 3:	Trial 3:	Trial 3:	Trial 3:	Trial 3:

At the end of this chapter, we include a list of some additional exposures to bodily sensations that may be relevant or helpful, depending on what types of symptoms alarm you. These are not core exposures we practice with everyone, but might be helpful for you in mimicking the sensations that alarm you.

As with all exposures, ensure that you practice interoceptive exposures in a variety of situations, and often. Do not practice them only when you are feeling at your best. Obviously, you can refrain if you are severely ill or your doctor has instructed you otherwise. However, patients will sometimes say they did not do the exposures because they were not in a good mood or were having some minor symptoms (e.g., a mild cold) and did not want to worsen their symptoms. Unless a doctor has told you to refrain from the behaviors outlined in the interoceptive exposures, we encourage you to do them regardless of whether you are feeling your best. Most people with illness anxiety worry about routine sensations, and therefore are most likely to get anxious when they notice normal symptoms or aren't in their best mood! Practicing in these situations can help make you more ready to tolerate sensations when you are not feeling your best.

Note that the exposures do not have to be highly distressing, or distressing at all, to be beneficial. It is most important that you are practicing bringing on bodily sensations and practicing tolerating them without trying to fight them off or figure out the cause of them. You may have mild to no anxiety when they you do the interoceptives, as the sensations may not bother you as much because you know the cause of the sensations and chose to induce them. If that is the case for you, that's fine! We still encourage you do all the interoceptive exposures. They still serve to get you more familiar with weird new sensations and teach you brain that these sensations are not always meaningful. Even if you recognize this on an intellectual level, anxious brains tend to not really learn this information until there is lived experience of having a lot of weird new sensations that are uneventful and not responded to with thoughts of "Ooh no! What is that?! Surely that is a sign of something serious ...." Rather, we can practice thinking, "I don't have to do anything about this sensation."

Eventually, combining interoceptive exposures with real-world exposure can be a great way to practice tolerating uncertainty of where the sensations are coming from and what they might mean. This tends to look different for everyone; therefore, we provide a case example below to demonstrate what combining some exposures may look like for one individual.

Example of a Patient Completing Interoceptive Exposures

Anne is a 33-year-old woman who has found that she has been worrying for months about potentially having an esophageal tumor. Across the months of her worry, she has noticed that she has intense periods of anxiety every time she notices a new, odd bodily sensation that wasn't there before, such as a feeling that she is not able to fully swallow, and a couple of times when she reported tasting blood in her mouth (although she did not see anything bleeding). Lately, she has been feeling a "bump in her chest," on a daily basis. She recently called her doctor to make an appointment to discuss this, but her physician scheduled an appointment with her for a month later, and did not seem to be in a rush to get her in based on her symptom report. She has been having difficulty tolerating the uncertainty that her physical symptoms might be signs of cancer. In addition, she has noticed that nearly every new sensation that arises, if it is more than mild and/or unfamiliar, she tends to attribute to the potential of having an esophageal tumor.

Anne sat down and developed an exposure hierarchy to target her fears of physical sensations that might be a sign of an esophageal tumor. She drafted the following hierarchy to target some specific sensations that she has feared lately, and some related ones that may arise. (Note that not all the exposures that she did are included, but below we focus on interoceptive-type exposures and interoceptive exposures combined with real-world exposures to give you an example.).

Anne's Mini-hierarchy to Target Fears of Physical Sensations Being a Sign of Esophageal Cancer

My exposure hierarchy	Anticipated SUDS (0–100)
Not drinking water for 20 minutes to feel a dry throat	25
Having a cough drop to maybe induce feeling of a lump in my throat	30
Breathing with open mouth for 5 minutes to induce dry mouth	35
Eating two crackers with no water for 10 minutes	40
Eating a sharp food (e.g., tortilla chip) that may cause me to feel like I have a small cut inside my mouth	45
Flossing (I know this will cause my gums to bleed slightly) to taste blood	50
Using a clean diabetes needle to give myself a tiny self-puncture on finger to have mild taste of blood in mouth	60
Cracker challenge—eating as many crackers as I can without water	70
Combining 5 minutes of mouth breathing, no water for an hour, 4 crackers, and eating something spicy	85
Combining mouth breathing, no water for an hour, 8 crackers eaten at my own pace, eating something spicy and describing the uncomfortable feeling in my stomach and bowels at the food passes through	100

Anne completed her exposure hierarchy across the course of three months, and successfully got more used to these sensations as she practiced them repeatedly. She reported that over the course of her practice, her final SUDS ratings for all the exposure items were around 4 or 5.

At the end of treatment, Anne reported that she still noticed signs that would have previously alarmed her, such as occasionally tasting blood in her mouth or heartburn after eating a lot of food or spicy food, but noted that she found these sensations slightly less alarming. She also noted that while her initial response to these sensations was still "Uh-oh!", she was quickly able to recognize that her anxiety was talking, and not engage in protective behaviors or prolonged worry about the symptoms.

Some Additional Interoceptive Exposure Examples

Lumps and Bumps
Wear clothing that creates excess skin "spillage" and creates the looks of lumps and bumps. Or feel your body for naturally existing compressions or dips (but make sure you do not complete safety behaviors in response to what you find).

Digestive Issues
Employ high-fiber foods or higher volumes of foods with high water content (e.g., grapes, watermelon) to create a feeling of fullness or bloat.

Irregularities on the Skin
Use cream that has a rough texture and feeling resembling these irregularities on your skin on purpose. You may want to do this while actively wishing for them to be medically problematic!

Cough/trouble Breathing
Wear a scarf over your head to cover your mouth while breathing, or exercise with a surgical mask on. Spend time in a sauna (where some people say it feels difficult to breathe). Eat foods that cause a tickle in your throat (e.g., drinking carbonated liquids at fast pace).

Throat Tightness/closing
Wear a tight scarf on your neck. Breathe in and out quickly to achieve a dry throat, then talk for five minutes without a drink of water. Or eat several saltine crackers without water and breathe through your mouth. Swallow food with a dry throat to have an internal feeling of lumps and bumps.

"Crackled" or Irregular Breathing
Wear a waist cincher to decrease breathing volume and increase feelings of suffocation. Complete a series of neti pot rounds to feel and hear crackling in the upper respiratory system (this can happen even without being congested). Breathe directly into a freezer.

Body Temperatures Slightly Above or Below Normal

Take baths/showers in colder and warmer water. Use your car's air conditioning and heater to rapidly change temperatures. Wear weather-inappropriate clothing to decrease your sensitivity—for example, wearing shorts on a semi-cold day or a sweater on a hot day.

Uncontrolled, Infrequent Body Movements (e.g., Eye Spasms)

Deliberately blinking your eyes at a rapid pace, or making movements on purpose that mimic the uncontrolled movements.

Pain (e.g., from Exercise, Aging, Accident, or Normal "Wear and Tear")

Complete a body scan in which the purpose is to identify areas of pain in the body and to fully observe and describe them without positive or negative judgement. Once those areas have been identified, move the body in slight, manageable ways to slightly increase the pain (the purpose is to not create more pain, but to accept and confront existing pain with the goal of tolerating it better).

Fatigue/tiredness

Stay up later and get up earlier to confront the feeling of being exhausted. Exercise more intensively to feel more low-energy. Have dry air blowing gently in your eyes (e.g., from a car vent), which can also lead to a feeling of dry or heavy eyes/tiredness.

Jitteriness/restlessness

Have one more cup of caffeinated coffee or tea than you usually do.

Changes in Menstruation

These may differ depending on the specific menstrual concern. Some examples are deliberately not keeping track of how long your cycle is or when you are due (while taking proper birth control cautions, if needed), or using tampons or maxi-pads that have too little or too much absorbency.

Visual Disturbances/changes

Press on your eyes with mild pressure (not excessively) to create floating clouds, bubbles, and spots in your vision.

Unexplainable "Unwell" Feeling (Malaise)

Eat foods that cause you to have a slight stomach upset or that are disgusting to you. You may want to do this along with exposures that target change in body temperatures (see above).

Explainable but Uncomfortable Age-related Changes

Examples might include, hair thinning, wrinkles, or more changes in the skin. You can draw more wrinkles on yourself, do a fun and anxiety-provoking make-up tutorial for aging skin, or use an aging app on you smartphone.

8

Imaginal Exposures

Check-in on Treatment Homework

Thought-challenging Practice

It's extremely important to do the treatment homework if you want to improve your anxiety symptoms, which is why westart every chapter by checking in on how you have been doing with the practice. First, let's check in on the thought-challenging. Have you been using the Thought-challenging Form to examine your thoughts every time you notice an upswing in distress related to health? If you have not been doing the challenging regularly, use the form now to go through some examples retrospectively. Doing this retrospectively is certainly not ideal, as our memory and thoughts tend to distort over time, but it is better to do some thought-challenging than none! So work through any examples of notable illness anxiety you noticed over the past week, and add to the form any you haven't challenged yet.

Sometimes patients are reluctant to stop and fill out the form during the week, and cite a variety of reasons. We highly encourage you to do the form formally, taking the time to self-reflect and make thoughtful written challenges. For most people, this takes time and effort. Below are some of the most common excuses we hear for not completing the Thought-challenging Form, along with the reasons why we encourage you to do the Thought-challenging Form in written detail.

DOI: 10.4324/9781032711355-8

"I Didn't Get Time"

Realistically, the Thought-challenging Form shouldn't take most people more than minutes a day. However, do make sure that you take the time to diligently inventory thoughts and challenge them: don't rush through the exercise just to get it done, but carefully consider alternative thoughts. Practicing changing thoughts takes quite a bit of self-reflection. Ideally, the thought-challenging should be a tool in the moment to slightly reduce your anxiety when you notice a peak of it. Sometimes when illness anxiety thoughts are high and worth challenging, people are involved in other things (e.g., driving, business meetings) that are incompatible with using the monitoring form. We suggest that, when possible, you do the challenging as soon after as possible. Some people keep a copy of the monitoring form on their bedside table or something similar, so that they remember to challenge anything that they did not get a chance to work through that day, at the very least.

"I Do It in My Mind Anyway"

You might feel that you are doing the thought-challenging fully enough in your mind, so why bother to go through the rigmarole of writing it all down? While mentally challenging is better than nothing, we highly encourage you to write it down. There is definitely an impact from getting your thoughts out of your head and seeing them on paper. While anxious thoughts often seem very real in our mind, people often tend to notice more distortions when they see their thoughts on paper. The paper can also serve as a log of previously challenged thoughts that can be helpful to add to and review periodically. Many patients have said that reviewing their prior thought-challenging logs gave them much insight into how their mind tends to get carried away with making predictions that are wildly catastrophic and unhelpful. Remember the well example, your insight into yourself is limited because we are limited when looking at ourselves. Completing these logs helps you take an objective look at yourself, as if you are your own therapist.

"It Might Make Me Feel Worse if I Pay Attention to Negative Thoughts"

Some people say that they are worried that if they write down or pay attention to their worries, they will spend more time thinking about them, that it will start them worrying or obsessing, or that the Thought-challenging Form will otherwise make their symptoms worse. This can absolutely happen if you believe these thoughts are true and if you do not use your skills. If you have thoughts like this, we encourage you to identify those as among the negative thoughts that arise with anxiety, and challenge them by looking for evidence and distortions, just like you would challenge other anxious thoughts.

"My Thoughts Seem True—I Couldn't Think of Any Challenges"

Make sure that you are writing down your interpretation of the situation, not just your emotions. Also make sure that you are asking yourself the "If that's true, what's so bad about that?" question and writing down any additional thoughts. A thought-monitoring log with "I feel frustrated. The doctor may have missed something" is hard to challenge. There certainly always is some chance that the doctor has missed something. However, the interpretations that led to the frustration, and the additional assumptions about the doctor missing something might be, for example: "I can't trust doctors," "Even if doctors say that I am fine I have to do my own research," "This happens every time I go to the doctor's," "They didn't look hard enough to know if I have cancer or not," and so on.

We include another Thought-challenging Form later in this chapter so that you can continue to practice thought-challenging this week.

If you did the challenging throughout the week, did you feel any better after you did it? Remember that in most cases, it should reduce distress at least slightly. If this is not the case, you may not be challenging what is most scary about the situation for you, or the real interpretations you are making. These can be hard to identify. Sometimes people get fairly skilled at challenging basic surface-level health-anxious fears, such as exaggerated estimates of serious health conditions. However, they might not be challenging some of the heavier implications that they are making to themselves that are typically much more difficult to identify. To practice digging down a couple layers to identify some of the core beliefs that drive some of the anxious fears, you may want to ask the "What's so bad about that?" question a couple of times. Remember the downward arrow from Chapter 2? If you don't, that's OK. It's simple: once you've identified an anxious fear, ask yourself: If that were true, why would that be so bad for me? What sense am I making of it? You can ask these questions again to identify additional beliefs. Often, these downward arrow "layers" are some of the most important beliefs to challenge! Remember, too, it is a commonplace experience to be able to logically challenge your thoughts, but still feel anxious about them for a while until exposure practice is done to test these thoughts thoroughly. Hopefully, though, the challenging will give you a bit more courage to do the exposures as you begin to see the mismatch between what you believe and what you feel.

Since identifying these additional interpretations can be quite difficult, to give you an idea of what this cognitive challenging process might look like, we provide some case examples below (fictional, but based on what we commonly see in practice).

Adrian, a 39-year-old graduate student, had worried for years about a variety of health conditions, but typically worried that he might develop diabetes. He remembered as a child watching his grandfather experience several complications related to his diabetes, and his grandfather always seemed miserable about his condition, saying, "I hope this never happens to you." Since childhood, Adrian had feared that he would also develop diabetes. While Adrian continued to feel that his chances of developing diabetes were relatively high, citing a family history of diabetes and some other risk factors such as being overweight and having a somewhat sedentary lifestyle, he was able to acknowledge the likelihood was much smaller than the chance that he would never develop diabetes. However, he reported that despite challenging these beliefs about likelihood, he continued to feel that

| I go to my annual physical that I have been avoiding | ⇒ | Doctor will tell me I am pre-diabetic or diabetic | ⇒ | I end up with diabetes complications: go blind, foot amputation | ⇒ | I've worked so hard and now I can't enjoy my life at all |

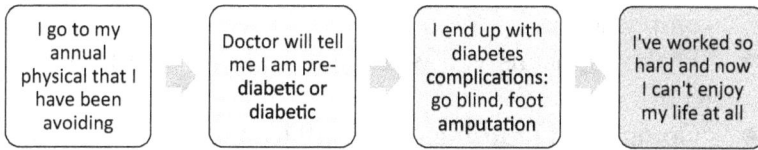

FIGURE 8.1 Downward arrow example 4

his ongoing anxiety about diabetes was excessive. He reported feeling that he continued to challenge the likelihood of developing diabetes over and over, but never felt any better, knowing it was always a possibility.

His therapist discussed with Adrian that while he appeared to be relatively good at practicing challenging overestimations of scary outcomes happening, he did not appear to be challenging the deeper interpretations that he was implying to himself about what having diabetes might mean or lead to. His therapist repeated the downward arrow process with him to get a better sense of these interpretations, asking "If that were true, what would be the worst part about that to you? What scares you the most about that?" to get at some additional fearful interpretations. Usually, the downward arrow works best with a situation you are avoiding or excessively protecting yourself against because of your fears, so Adrian and his therapist selected his avoidance of an annual check-up with his general practitioner that he had been putting off. The results of this process are shown in Figure 8.1.

Based on this, it became apparent to both Adrian and his therapist that there were more cognitive interpretations that could be challenged, as there are many implied assumptions in the chain of events Adrian was worried would happen. Together, they made a list of additional related thoughts to challenge, which Adrian was sent home with so that he could practice thinking of challenges for them. The list of assumptions/implications included:

◆ "If I go to my doctor's appointment, it is likely they will tell me I have diabetes or pre-diabetes."
◆ "If I am pre-diabetic, that means I will eventually have diabetes."

◆ "If I get diabetes, I will end up with significant medical complications."

◆ "Diabetes means you will likely go blind and lose your feet."

◆ "Going blind or losing a foot will lead to complete loss of enjoyment in life."

◆ "Having diabetes means you can't enjoy life."

Again, we do not mean to suggest that some of Adrian's feared outcomes are not negative or scary in ways, such as foot amputation. These deeper fears are also often more difficult to challenge than the more basic surface-level thoughts, because there is usually always some chance they will occur, just like many negative events in life. However, just like most anxious thoughts, people are generally overestimating how likely and severe these situations would be, and underestimating how well they would cope even if a negative scenario occurred.

Laren, a 38-year-old high-powered environmental lawyer, had been worried for years that she might develop breast cancer. She reported having several family members and friends who had received a diagnosis of breast cancer, and noted that she lost two close family members to cancer. She reported that in the past she had undergone a series of tests when her physician was unsure whether she might have cancer or not, and found the process distressing and extremely disruptive to her life. She reported that now, nearly each time she noticed nearly any physical symptom (e.g., fever, stomach upset), she worried it might be a sign of cancer. She could acknowledge that she likely catastrophized and overestimated the likelihood of negative things happening. In fact, she did some basic research about incidence rates of breast cancer in people like her and learned from reputable sources that she was dramatically overestimating the chances she would get cancer. She was also aware that there are hundreds of things that may be considered "signs" of various forms cancer, and how easy it is to interpret any new symptom as a potential sign of cancer, given the high rates of lay theories on the internet. However,

Schedule appointments during times of important work events	I get bad or ambiguous news (e.g., "more tests needed")	I will be too focused on the uncertainty to concentrate	I say something offensive or factually wrong	I'm not trusted in my field and never hired again

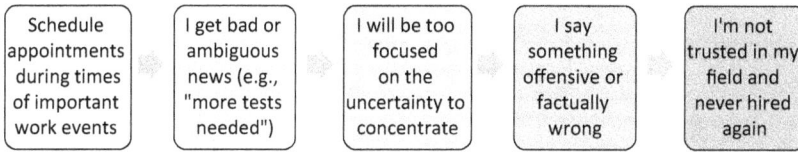

FIGURE 8.2 Downward arrow example 5

she continued to report experiencing days of excessive rumination when she noticed any new symptom. Laren did the downward arrow shown in Figure 8.2 with her avoidance behavior, which was avoiding scheduling important work projects (such as important meetings or talks) around the times when she scheduled medical appointments.

Just like Adrian, Laren had many assumptions embedded in her downward arrow that were challengeable. Some of her example challenges are listed below to give you a sense of how she used her Thought-challenging Form to look at the evidence to ensure she was thinking about her fears in a factual way and not basing her conclusions on emotions or early assumptions.

Anxious interpretation	What distortions are present? What are the facts? Re-write your thoughts without distortions.
If I get bad or ambiguous medical news, I will have such trouble concentrating at work, and it will lead to serious mistakes or saying something offensive.	I am fortune telling here. I have had trouble concentrating at work in the past when I am anxious, but I was still able to do my job, even though I felt worried nearly all the time. While I definitely feel I didn't perform at my best, it never led to a mistake I couldn't come back from.
If I say something factually wrong, I will not be trusted in my field.	This is fortune telling again, and not accurate, as I have definitely said things that were not factually true in the past! Sometimes people noticed, but mostly not—and it never led to serious repercussions. I have decades of hard work and achievement to point to to prove I am capable in my field even if I make a mistake.

Anxious interpretation	*What distortions are present? What are the facts? Re-write your thoughts without distortions.*
Saying something wrong or offensive at work will lead to my not being hired anywhere again.	I *feel* that others will judge me negatively, as I have seen my coworkers judge others negatively at times, but I don't know for sure what they will think. It's possible my great track record would outweigh most mistakes. I'm pretty sure that even if I lost this job, I could find another in the field.
It is important to always be on point at work and never distracted, otherwise you can make a mistake with serious consequences.	I do think it is important to be on point at work, but "never distracted" is impossible. Most people go through things at various points in their lives that take up a lot of their mental space—such as divorce, loss, financial problems, etc. I know they often still go to work and function, and it's OK if they think about those things at times—that's just human nature.

Thought-challenging Form

Trigger (What started the anxiety? Or what was going on at the time when you noticed your anxiety spike?)	Thoughts (Then, if that thought were true, what would be so bad about that?)	What distortions are present? What are the facts? Re-write your thoughts without distortions.

Exposure Practice

Let's also check in again on how you have been doing with the exposures. Have you been doing daily practice of the exposure you selected in the last chapter? Did you practice that exercise for at least a week? Has your anxiety about the exposure situation reduced? If not, you may want to revisit some of the problem-solving about exposures in Chapter 6. We generally suggest continued frequent practice until your SUDS rating is in the 30s or lower.

Below is another exposure form to select and track the next exposure that you will do next week. Most people do the next exposure on their hierarchy, but if you are feeling quite confident that you can refrain from safety behaviors and go higher, go ahead! Usually at this point, people are doing exposure items from their hierarchy that they initially rated around a SUDS level of 50–60.

This week's exposure(s):

Anticipated discomfort (SUDS)	My anxious predictions: What do I think will happen when I do this (e.g., will I get hurt, ill, or die)? How uncomfortable will I be, and for how long?	Actual SUDS the final time I did the task this week	Actual outcome

Imaginal Exposures

We discussed in the prior chapter that sometimes there are health anxiety worries involving anxious predictions made so far in advance that they are not immediately testable or knowable. Some examples again are:

> "Someday I will get cancer and be in pain and hospice for several years."
> "If I get Hepatitis, I will not be able to enjoy life."
> "I will be terrified when I am dying alone."

While these certainly often reflect worries that are exaggerated just like other health anxious worries, for the most part they are not immediately testable. In these cases, one option is to do imaginal exposures.

Imaginal exposure involves practicing having unwanted thoughts, memories, or imagery in order to learn that these internal experiences are not as dangerous as they feel. It means intentionally thinking the very things that scare you the most, in a prolonged, systematic way. This generally entails writing out your personal "horror story"—the details of your feared outcomes that would make them so scary for you, and spending time thinking about them in lots of detail. Imaginal exposure has been used for decades as an integral part of the cognitive behavioral treatment for many anxiety and related disorders, and appears to have benefits for factors such as ability to tolerate uncertainty, worry, and depressed mood.[1-4] Imaginal exposure can also often be a helpful first step in beginning to approach a feared situation if it feels particularly daunting. It can often feel easier to practice approaching a feared thought than a feared situation or outcome, especially if you are having a very difficult time completing a real-world exposure.

Intentionally thinking about your fears may immediately seem paradoxical to you, as you might think, "I worry about my feared outcomes all the time, and I'm still anxious!" There are some key differences in your regular worry versus doing intentional imaginal exposures. First, in doing the imaginal exposure exercises, the point is that you want to think carefully about the feared outcomes that scare you, and sit with that imagery and feeling for a prolonged period, just like when doing a real-world exposure (like those from your hierarchy). Just like real-world exposure, sitting with these mental experiences for a prolonged period can lead to some habituation—getting more used to the idea of the scary outcome, or at least taking some of the edge off. Second, part of the imaginal exposure is learning to practice tolerating an emotional state: usually the discomfort of uncertainty. When we worry outside of imaginal exposures, but most people try to fight the worries, images, or feelings off. We might also try to protect ourselves by convincing ourselves we are or will be OK, or jump from aspect to aspect or worry to worry. We typically do not stick with a scenario and think it through thoroughly, from beginning to end, with all the implied sequelae. Doing so can help us see that some of our predictions may be unfounded, but also, you can get more used to tolerating that feeling of discomfort that comes from not knowing. Sitting with that feeling is the point of the exposure! Finally, imaginal exposure is under your control. By electing to voluntarily approach your worries and stand your ground, you can get a sense of mastery and control over your fears and potentially feel less like they bully you around.

Imaginal Exposure as a First or Intermediary Step in Exposure

If you are still having a hard time doing exposures as planned, imaginal exposure can sometimes be an intermediary step that gets you closer to the actual exposure. To illustrate this clearly, we will use an example unrelated to illness anxiety: someone who is highly afraid of dogs. Imagine that you had an intense fear of dogs (assuming you do not already), and that you began cognitive behavioral treatment for this fear. If we set out to practice exposure and immediately suggested that you go to a dog park to play with a bunch of dogs, you would likely say no way! Even though being able to be around a dog or even playing with a dog might be an end goal in treatment, it would likely feel too scary to immediately try this high-level exposure when you are just beginning exposures. The chances of your agreeing to an activity like this would be slim. An easier starting place might be to think about (imagine) the last time you saw a dog. Likely this would yield less anxiety than being around an actual dog. We might also start to think about the fears related to being around dogs, such as, "I might get bitten."

Imaginal exposures can also be quite helpful when you are unable to design exposures to your feared outcome. In the above dog phobia example, we would never do exposure to actually getting bitten by a dog just so you could learn that you could tolerate it and that it was not as bad as anticipated. That would not be ethical or helpful. We might instead do an imaginal exposure to the scary thought "I might get bitten" or "I can't be sure if I will get bitten." Later in this chapter we will give some examples of how to begin practicing this. Using an example more related to illness anxiety, we would not do something like try to give you cancer intentionally just to show you that you can tolerate it better than expected, and that the cancer experience is different than anticipated. However, we can think through your scary "cancer story" in detail, looking for accuracies and inaccuracies, and facing feared outcomes and thoughts over and over again until they lose some of their bite.

Exposure to Uncertainty

One element that is almost always emphasized in health anxiety imaginal exposures is the idea of uncertainty. The health anxiety worries discussed at the start of this chapter each share a common theme when examined closely: uncertainty about an outcome in the future that is not immediately knowable. We cannot know if someday we will get cancer. We cannot know for sure if we will contract hepatitis. We cannot know how we will feel when we will die or if we will die alone. We coexist each day with a great variety of uncertainties.

It is normal and human to have some fear related to the unknown. This fear has likely been selected as an evolutionary advantage for humans over the course of time as it has helped keep humans safe to some degree. However, for some anxious people, uncertainty feels particularly intolerable and triggers attempts to avoid or resolve uncertainty as much as possible. In illness anxiety, you likely know by now that this can present as anxious health behaviors (such as excessive reassurance-seeking, mental checking or reviewing, internet research, etc.). However, for the most part, even after engaging in one of these behaviors, we are still left with uncertainty. These behaviors are rarely able to give us the certainty we desire, although they may give the brief illusion of it. These behaviors often give us some sense of relief, which is why they are continued, but the relief tends to be temporary, as real certainty cannot be had. Moreover, these behaviors serve to fuel the body's fear or intolerance of uncertainty. In reality, we cannot be sure about many health-related outcomes, and this is a reality we need to face.

Look at Figure 8.3, which shows an example of this anxious cycle. You can see that at the core of each sample avoidant behavior (body checking, reassurance-seeking, mental checking, and review) is a health fear—in our example, fear of possibly getting cancer one day. The avoidant behaviors of body checking serve to distract temporarily from the fear of uncertainty about one

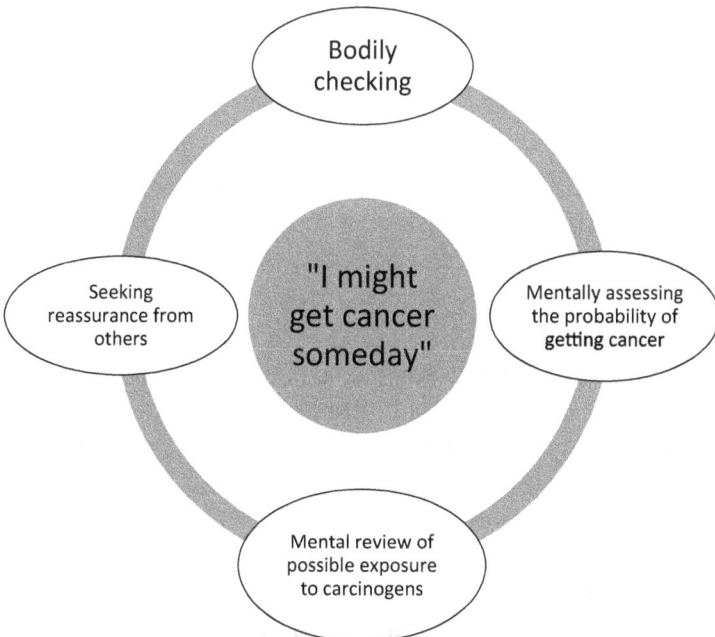

FIGURE 8.3 Cancer concern example

day developing cancer. In imaginal exposure, we want you to do the opposite: focus on the feared thought (e.g., "I might get cancer someday") without distracting with mental activity, seeking reassurance, or checking. Just like with other forms of exposure, the more you focus on the fear in the moment, the more comfortable with it you will get in time. In doing this, you will also collect important data on your own ability to tolerate and cope with the emotional experience of uncertainty.

Some people hear about imaginal exposures and ask, "Wwhy would I want to think about or tell myself such negative things? Don't I want to tell myself I won't get cancer?" This is a fair question. It can also be confusing if you have been practicing the cognitive challenging, as many people are trying to do some talking back to their overestimations of likelihood by saying "This scary health outcome isn't as likely as I feel it is." Patients may become confused and ask "What am I supposed to say to myself when I am anxious?" The advice is quite simple: be honest with yourself. That scary health outcome it is not as likely as you think it is, but you do have to coexist with the fact that your feared outcome is always possible.

In this example, it likely feels much more pleasant to tell yourself that you will not contract cancer one day. Our guess is that you have already tried this. If you are reading this workbook, we would assume that this strategy has not been helpful so far. It is likely that when you told yourself "I won't get cancer," anxiety popped up in the back of your mind and asked, "Can you be sure about that?", and the cycle of avoidant behaviors and resultant anxiety continued. When it comes to imaginal exposure, honesty is the best policy. We cannot know for sure whether you will get cancer someday. Though it is scarier to focus on that unknown, it has the benefit of truth—this is not knowable right now, and no amount of checking, mental review, etc. is going to let you know something that is unknowable.

A concept we frequently discuss in our treatment of health anxiety is "self-efficacy." This concept is similar to self-confidence, and refers to our ability to know that when we are faced with something difficult, we have skills on our own that we can securely and confidently depend on to get us through successfully. This concept is fully applicable in terms of tolerating uncertainty. We like to remind our patients of ways they are already self-efficacious in tolerating uncertainty in their lives currently. For example, most of drive—despite full awareness that we could get in a car accident. We enter relationships despite not knowing whether they will last, work out, or backfire. We ask: do they need to know exactly how their Monday work day will go, or can they tolerate changes in their schedule if they happen? If they forgot a meeting, would they be able to move other scheduled items around to accommodate? Sure, it may not be ideal, but they would be able to do it. You already tolerate uncertainty in most areas of your life, and can use those experiences to realize that you already have skills, and just need to generalize them (or apply) them to your health anxiety. It's not reinventing the wheel, but saying, "How can I use my current wheel/system in this new issue or concern?"

We also do imaginal exposures to counteract the harmful effects of thought suppression, which is when people try to avoid thinking about things that bother them or avoid having related negative feelings. As mentioned in previous chapters, we know that the more you tries to suppress your thoughts, the more of those thoughts you will likely have. Use the following exercise right now look at an object in front of you. Focus on that object for 30 seconds. Time yourself. Now think of anything and everything you can to focus away from that object, think about anything but that object. Is all you can think about that object? This the same thing as thinking about an elephant in your room. OK, now do whatever you have to in order *not to* think about the elephant. Is the elephant all you can think about now? Well, you aren't alone! You are likely doing the same thing with your thoughts about your health anxiety. The more we tell ourselves to *not* think about something, the more the thought stays present, and even increases. Allowing the thought to be present ends this cycle of struggle with the anxiety bully.

Sample Imaginal Exposures

It can be difficult to know how thorough to be with an imaginal exposure, or what exactly to include in it. Therefore, we provide some examples of imaginal exposure narratives below. These examples do not come from any particular patient (to protect confidentiality), but rather are fictional but realistic examples of themes we commonly hear.

Patients are often unsure how much detail or what kind of content should be included. The short answer is there is no ideal length. The type of content depends on what makes you feel anxious: the imaginal exposure narrative should focus on the very themes that make you feel anxious, and include a detailed description of the sequelae of those happenings. Use your imagination to fill in details. The more vividly you can imagine the scenario, the better. For example, in this fictional scenario, what exactly did the doctor say to you? How did you feel inside when they said it? Were there any sights, sounds, smells that increased your anxiety? Some people even go into the temperature, time of day, etc. Describe your feared scenario in play-by-play chronological detail that is so vivid anyone could read it and put themselves in those shoes. The more you can make your experience whole, the more realistic and effective an exposure it will be for you.

Lower-level imaginal exposures may be shorter and may focus on a single negative aspect of the feared situation, and not go much beyond that. In the later stages of treatment, we will typically ensure that the exposure narratives really detail the sequelae of the feared outcome, asking, "What happens then? If that occurs, what next?"

If patients are very unsure what their imagined outcomes may look like, or are concluding that their perception of the actual experience may be way off, we often have them do some brief research to get a sense of what it may entail. For example, if they feel excessively anxious about the physical discomfort that may arise from chemotherapy, but feel somewhat unsure about what the process looks like or what physical sensations might be expected, we may have them read or watch videos of first-hand stories about experiences with chemotherapy, or read a brief article online describing what the treatment looks like. Getting these details can make the imaginal picture more vivid and simultaneously serve as an exposure that often corrects misconceptions about feared situations. Therefore, collecting some brief information about what your feared scenario may look like is often not a bad choice if you are unsure what it may entail, and if you are careful not to use it as a safety behavior (e.g., to over-research it so that you can reassure yourself you would be able to tolerate it, or to convince yourself it won't happen).

Imaginal Exposure Example 1: Missing Potential Cancer Signs

The first example imaginal exposure narrative below reflects a patient, *Anna*, who is very anxious about responding quickly to medical signs and symptoms she notices. She lives by the motto "early detection saves lives," and has a great fear of cancer reoccurrence despite being in full remission for several years. She therefore checks her body daily for signs and symptoms, and frequently requests extra medical testing despite being told by her physicians that check-ins twice per year are adequate. Because her fear surrounds what would happen if she did not maintain high vigilance to her body and catch signs early, her exposure narrative surrounds what would happen if she did not catch signs and diligently report them to her doctor. It also emphasizes elements that might heighten her anxiety, such as the doctor appearing unsure or incompetent, fear of discomfort from chemotherapy, and elements of uncertainty.

> *I'm waiting six months to go back in for a medical recheck, like my doctor suggested. In the second month, I start to notice breast soreness on some days. When I touch my breast, I feel something that might be a lump—I can't tell. I think my therapist would suggest that I wait and follow my medical doctor's advice, and I just had a scan, so I don't do anything.*
>
> *When I go back to the doctor for my appointment in six months, I tell her about what I've noticed. She says she's concerned and recommends that we get more testing done, at least a biopsy. The doctor mumbles some reservations about why we waited so long for a recheck, and she seems to be taking a lot of time to try to figure out what to do, seeming unsure about what testing is best. I feel like for sure it's going to be something bad.*
>
> *With the next round of testing, they tell me that the biopsy has determined that the thing that felt like a lump is cancer. They*

mention that it got worse rapidly; they ask, "Why didn't you come in earlier?" They tell me I need to choose between surgery and chemo, or both. I am weighing the huge amount of information they gave me, the statistics, side effects, probabilities, I feel so overwhelmed and unsure of what is the best decision. I end up choosing chemo after weighing it out. They tell me they are going to intravenously put chemicals into my body.

When I get the chemo, throughout those weeks I feel sick almost every day. I am nauseous and vomiting, and gradually lose hair. I can't stop thinking about how there's a cancer in my body—a foreign invader I can do nothing about. I'm puking almost every day for three months, and I avoid going out because I feel sick most of the time.

After several weeks of chemo treatment, the doctor has a meeting with me to tell me the chemo isn't really working, and that death is likely at some point in the next year. I think: this is unfair. I'm young. This is not how I envisioned my life to go. I'm going to miss out on tons of stuff with my kids and husband: I will never know what my kids choose to do for their careers, I will not be able to go traveling with my husband, there are many fun things I will never do. I probably could have caught the cancer earlier if I had just gone into the doctor. I should have known from the sensations and done something: I made a huge mistake.

Imaginal Exposure Example 2: Worry about the Health of Others

When people have illness anxiety, they most often worry about their personal health. However, given that they are often over-vigilant to health signs and have heightened beliefs about control and responsibility, excessive health fears may also spill over to family members. Therefore, below we offer an example of imaginal exposure for excessive worry regarding a family member. This (fictional) patient, *Hannah*, attempts to stay over-vigilant about her mother's health after a cancer scare, and for years has been trying to research and persuade her mother to make specific heath decisions, despite her mother being capable of making competent heath decisions for herself. She particularly worries about her mother not disclosing information to her.

Mom continues to see her doctor for regular follow-ups to ensure that her cancer says in remission. Checking in with her, my brother and I start to notice that mom is mentioning that the doctor is recommending getting scans/procedures, but that she is not scheduling these or talking about them with us as she usually does. I haven't seen her in a while. When I finally see her, she is pale, tired, and looks like she has lost a lot of weight. She calls me after I leave her house and says, 'Look, I have to tell you something.' She says, 'They found cancer again. It is advanced, and while there are some treatments that have been recommended, I do not want to go through more procedures about it.' She tells me there is a lot more that she has not told me until now, and has been keeping things from me for a while so as not to make me more anxious. I had told myself this was an irrational thought all along, and now it turned out to be true. She chose less time with us and things she wanted to do, and there is nothing I can do about it. I realize that there is a whole new process to manage now: what will happen with mom? I think about having to make end-of-life decisions for her, although I know she has planned all of these things already.

Once you have written your imaginal exposure narrative, make sure to set aside time to read it for at least 15 minutes a day, imagining it in detail and allowing yourself to feel any emotions that arise without trying to fight them off. Focus on the very parts about it that spike up your anxiety and uncertainty.

Advanced Topic: Is Illness Anxiety Simply a Fear of Death?

When patients with illness anxiety first contact our clinic for treatment, it is not uncommon for them to report that the problem for which they are seeking treatment is "fear of dying." While completing treatment, they may ask, "Isn't illness anxiety just a fear of death?"

While death and dying are certainly major themes that come up in treating illness anxiety, we tend to not conceptualize illness anxiety as simply a fear of death. Fear of death is not necessarily pathological—some fear of death is normal and appropriate in human beings! Being afraid of danger and dying is an evolutionarily adaptive trait that likely helped keep our ancestors alive. Individuals who were more anxious about dying were likely more avoidant of dangerous situations and took fewer risks, making it more likely that they remained alive and reproduced. Their children were likely to inherit those genes that predisposed them to some level of cautiousness. Therefore, it's likely that there was some genetic selection for individuals who were anxious enough to avoid danger and take some precautions. In today's world, fear of death continues to serve to motivate us in a similar way: to avoid taking excessive risks and to drive us to take natural health and safety precautions. As clinicians treating anxiety, we would never try to *remove* death anxiety from a patient, even if we could. In short, in many ways it is a protective and adaptive thing, although it can be uncomfortable, like many adaptive emotions are.

Secondly, in illness anxiety, excessive worries tend to specifically surround fears of dying via illness or other health-related problems. The person with illness anxiety often has a comparative lack of similarly intense fears about other ways of dying that may on the surface seem quite similar in terms of catastrophic outcomes, suddenness, pain, family impact, or likelihood. For example, patients may acknowledge that they ruminate most of the day about a sudden death from an aneurysm, but do not worry as excessively about sudden death from other catastrophes such as car crashes, attacks, or other catastrophic incidents. Therefore, literal death does not seem to be the primary anxiety driver, but rather dying in a certain way, or some part of the process of illness and dying. While some people may certainly be afraid of themes related to death, such as uncertainty about whether there is an afterlife, usually they are afraid of themes that are more specific to medical illness, such as loss of control, or an exaggerated sense of personal responsibility to prevent bad outcomes.

This is why the downward arrow is particularly important: it helps to identify *what about* having an illness, or what about the dying process, is so scary for you. Different people can be concerned with different parts of the process of illness and death. For example, some people may say, "I'm not afraid of dying, but rather the prolonged pain and suffering before," or "the idea that I could have prevented it and didn't," and so on. Identifying what your personal fears are with downward arrow can make them easier to challenge, and potentially easier to design exposures to.

Just like all anxious cognitions, we are often overestimating how bad feared situations are. We are often imagining the process of dying in many ways that do not match the experiences we hear from people who are in the process of dying.

So take a moment to think about it now: do you think you may have exaggerated negative beliefs about the badness of dying? Take a moment to really think about it, and write down your responses below. Make sure to think about it carefully and write down your fears as well as possible so that they can be challenged in the next section.

What are you specifically worried about when it comes to death and dying? Are you afraid of death, or are you afraid of something else about the process of serious or sudden illness, such as suffering, loss, or lack of control. And even if you suffer some, regret some, or have some lack of control, why is that so bad to you? What does that mean about you or the world? What are you telling yourself about what you think it will be like?

_____

_____

_____

_____

_____

_____

_____

_____

_____

Now use your thought-challenging skills to challenge your thoughts about death and dying. Do you see any of the cognitive distortions present in any of your thoughts? For example, are you making potentially catastrophic predictions without much evidence to bet on that outcome? Are you saying "I shoulds," "oughts," or "have tos" to yourself?

Include these thoughts on your Thought-challenging Form for the week, and practice challenging them just as you would any other negative thoughts you are having related to your illness anxiety. Below are some example entries to give you some idea of what this might look like.

Thought-Challenging Form (Example)

Thoughts (Then, if that thought were true, what would be so bad about that?)	What distortions are present? What are the facts? Re-write your thoughts without distortions.
If I die suddenly, my sons will grow up without me. They will never recover from the loss. The experience will be traumatic for them, and they will not be as successful in life as they could have been.	This is me fortune telling and projecting my feelings and fears onto them. While I was devastated by the loss of my grandmother, I do not know they would experience a death similarly. They seem to cope with things well. While I think it would definitely impact them, it may impact them less than I think. Knowing them, I predict that they will be sad occasionally, but will still be able to move forward in life.
I will live with a cancer diagnosis for at least a year knowing that I am going to die, in terrible physical pain and continuous depression.	This is fortune telling. While getting a fatal cancer diagnosis would be very sad and I would be anxious at times, I do not know how it would impact me. I have watched a lot of videos online of people with cancer, and after a period of adjustment, many of them seemed to cope with it remarkably well. I honestly do not know what kind of pain would be involved and for how long. I have heard many cancer patients (on TV and from articles about them) say that they have "good days and bad days."

Next, let's talk about related exposures. Since many death-related processes are things we cannot realistically (or ethically!) create real-world exposures for, these are usually great themes to do imaginal exposures with. Write out a script that details your own death, and that emphasizes what about the process for you would be so scary. Remember that these are often high-level exposures for people, so they often trigger lots of emotions—sadness, guilt, anxiety, and so on. That's OK! Remember that part of doing these exposures is to allow yourself to feel emotions rather than fighting them off excessively. The emotions will pass in their own due time, and the less you try to fight them off, usually the less intense and impairing they are in the long run.

Note that you do not need to write a "sob story" to try to make yourself feel as bad as possible. We expect you to feel sad and have some nervousness about death—that is expected! The point is to emphasize what about the story makes you feel anxious and uncertain, particularly thoughts, images, or feelings you might be trying to avoid. Use the beliefs you identified above to highlight the parts that feel especially scary to you, adding as much imaginary detail as possible.

You can also watch movies or true stories where people were dying, facing death, or losing loved ones. You want to confront and expose yourself to the emotions related to death and find some acceptance and peace about it. You will never be OK with the thought of death. Even for those with a strong sense of faith and the afterlife, there is still some concern about the dying process. It is the ultimate unknown. You won't know it until you go through it.

Here is an example imaginal exposure narrative based on the example entry in the Thought-challenging Form above:

I have a sudden heart attack and die within a couple minutes. I did not see it coming—there were no signs or symptoms. It is so quick I do not even know I am dying; I have strong chest pain, and then suddenly I've lost consciousness. The police find my body in a car on the side of the road, as I was driving when it happened. Two uniformed police go to my house to inform my family. They knock on the door; my wife and sons are there.

They tell everyone to sit down. They say, "There is no easy way to inform you of this, but your husband was found deceased today in a car accident. It looks like it may have been a heart attack." My family immediately starts sobbing and is devastated. My wife is not sure how she will be able to live without me.

My sons grow up through their teen years. Throughout that time, my wife struggles to manage them, as she is not as good at discipline and structure as I was. The boys do not have a male influence in the home, and always resent not having a dad around. They feel that they stand out from other kids. They both turn into adults with anxiety and depression, and must see a therapist for most of their lives. They struggle to succeed in school. I know that I am not aware of it as I am deceased and not conscious any more, but I do not get to see any of their life milestones. I do not get to see their marriages, their achievements, their graduations. I am not there to support them, or to show them how to do things such as repairs, so they struggle. My wife often feels stressed and is hesitant to take on a new relationship as she was so traumatized from the loss. My entire family's life was negatively impacted by my death.

Once you have written your exposure narrative, give it a once-over to make sure you provided enough detail in areas you think are most associated with your anxiety. If there are images that particularly bother you, you may want to add detail about what these may look like. When complete, read the exposure narrative each day for at least 15 minutes, imagining it in detail and allowing yourself to feel the emotions that come up.

Religion, Spirituality, and Health Anxiety

The role of religion and spirituality in promoting or helping people to cope with illness anxiety has not been examined in detail. However, religious beliefs obviously have relevance when it comes to the core fears of patients with health anxiety and their related thoughts and feelings about death. Around 84% of the world's population identifies with some sort of religious affiliation.[5] The majority of organized religions in the world have philosophies and rites related to death, and associated concepts of afterlife or reincarnation. The existing research on how religion relates to anxiety is inconclusive, as there are many religionss, and unfortunately studies have used quite a variety of ways of measuring religion and spirituality, and in many types of groups of people. The findings have been conflictual, with some studies showing that religiosity (e.g., involvement with church peers, worship attendance, and practice) is associated with less anxiety, and some studies suggesting that certain religious beliefs and practices can be associated with increased risk for anxiety.[6]

Your religious beliefs may obviously help or hurt your anxiety, depending on the nature of them. If you currently have a religious faith, make sure to think about how it relates to your worries about your health. We find that many people we work with are ambivalent about their spiritual beliefs, not sure what to believe, or actively struggling with deciding what to believe in. While this workbook is not meant to push spirituality or any particular religion, you may want to consider looking into this part of your life more deeply if you feel it relates to your fears of illness anxiety and death. Some questions to consider, or to discuss with your therapist or religious leader you trust may include:

◆ How do you view illness and death in the context of religion and spirituality? How much do you believe these things—is your faith strong, moderate, weak?
◆ What would it mean to you to develop a deeper sense of spirituality or religion?
◆ How would developing your faith impact your health anxiety? What are the pros and cons?
◆ Can you seek out spiritual guidance to help you tolerate health anxiety? Would you seek out a spiritual guide, a shaman, a priest, rabbi? Is there anyone in your social support network (e.g., family, friends, partner, teacher) with whom you could explore this topic?

◆ Would you be able to be more flexible with yourself and your health if spirituality and religiosity were part of your life?

◆ A common theme in religion and spirituality is giving up your worldly concerns about your feared outcomes—that is, your health—to a higher power. How do you feel about this? How does this thought interact with your belief system?

9

Giving Healthcare an Appropriate Role in Your Life

Check-in on Treatment Homework

Thought-Challenging Practice

Have you been practicing challenging your negative thoughts when you have episodes of excessive anxiety? Are you finding that the anxious thoughts are less sticky in your brain? If you have been challenging similar thoughts by writing them down and challenging them daily, they should be getting easier to challenge, and people usually report some of the "edge" of anxiety has reduced.

If you have not found this to be the case, you may want to take another look at your Thought-challenging Form to make sure that you are challenging all the interpretations you are making. It is likely that there is a potentially meaty interpretation that you are implying to yourself about what the feared consequences mean about or the world, but that may not yet be identified. Be sure to challenge those thoughts as well! At this stage, most people are getting better at realizing they are overestimating how severe and likely their feared outcomes are. However, they are often not

DOI: 10.4324/9781032711355-9

challenging some of the deeper interpretations about themselves and the world they are telling themselves, for example about how they should always have control, how they should prepare for disaster to avoid disappointment, that they cannot trust doctors, that they are significantly more health fragile than others, and so on. Make sure this week you ask yourself the "What's so bad about that?" question and challenge those thoughts on the Thought-challenging Form as well. Below we have included another copy of the form for you to work on those thoughts.

Thought-challenging Form

Trigger (What started the anxiety? Or what was going on at the time when you noticed your anxiety spike?)	Thoughts (Then, if that thought were true, what would be so bad about that?)	What distortions are present? What are the facts? Re-write your thoughts without distortions.

Exposure Practice

Let's also check in again on how you have been doing with the exposures. Have you been doing daily practice of the exposure you selected in Chapter 8? Did you practice that exercise daily for at least a week? Has your anxiety about the exposure situation reduced? If not, you may want to revisit some of the problem-solving about exposures in Chapter 6. We generally suggest continued practice until your SUDS rating is in the 30s or lower.

Step back and look at all the exposures you have done already. Great job! You have taken some risks in challenging your anxious thoughts. What have you learned from the exposures you have done so far? How have the exposures felt, and what have the outcomes been compared with what you thought they would be like prior to doing them? Have you learned anything about your ability to tolerate distress and how long it hangs around? About whether you really need to do safety behaviors? Do you have enough evidence, or do you need more to feel confident in your conclusions?

Below is another exposure form to select and track the next exposure you will do next week. Most people do the next exposure level up on their hierarchy. Usually at this point, people are doing exposure items from their hierarchy that they initially rated around a SUDS level of 60–70.

This week's exposure(s):

Anticipated discomfort (SUDS)	My anxious predictions: What do I think will happen when I do this (e.g., will I get hurt, ill, or die)? How uncomfortable will I be, and for how long?	Actual SUDS the final time I did the task this week	Actual outcome

Also, how have you been doing with the imaginal exposure(s)? Were you able to read your imaginal exposure content daily and think about them in vivid detail, allowing yourself to feel any emotions that arose? If yes, great job—thinking about your worst-case scenario is a high-level exposure for many people.

If not, what got in the way? You've heard us say it before, but we'd like to reiterate that doing all of the exposures, including the imaginal exposures, is likely the most important part of the treatment. Doing them regularly, ideally daily, is often the best medicine for anxiety.

Moving Forward with Appropriate Health Behaviors

We recognize that for most people, some level of protective health behaviors is intrinsic to good health. We do not expect you to always refrain from things like medical research or appropriate preventative health behaviors. The problem is that individuals with illness anxiety often have trouble discerning between what is important and necessary versus what might be an unnecessary and anxiety-driving health behavior.

> *There is an appropriate amount of anxiety that people should have about the serious conditions they have. For example, 'I had a stroke; how do we make it not come back? How do we know if it happens again?' These are appropriate questions.*
>
> Dr. L., Internal Medicine

Many people report that they do not have a good sense of what is an appropriate amount of health behaviors! Often, they are basing their behavior off what they saw modeled for them growing up. Since anxiety disorders often have genetic and familial influences, it is common for individuals with illness anxiety to have grown up around a family member who was health-anxious, or to still have health-anxious people in their lives. Sometimes we have been doing health-protective behaviors for so long, or have seen those close to us do them, that we do not realize that the average person may be doing things quite differently! We have found that it is also common for individuals with illness anxiety to have someone in their vicinity—family member, spouse, or friend—who is also health-anxious and/or who spends a lot of time talking about or inquiring about health.

Another potentially pernicious influence can be a friend or family member who works in a human services or health profession, especially if you talk with them frequently about health-related issues. While individuals in healthcare professions are often extremely knowledgeable about their areas, they also often get filtered information that you are more likely to interpret catastrophically. For example, a nurse who works in an emergency room sees catastrophic injuries or illnesses on a regular basis, making it seem like they are much more common and disastrous than they actually are for most of the population. Also, they often go through intense training and education about their fields, hearing about the dangers of under-caution. For example, nurses are often trained day in and day out to carefully wash their hands, wear protective equipment, and so, to prevent deadly infections. While these habits are generally good in the workplace, they can overgeneralize outside the workplace or become overly rigid rules. Therefore, unless they are extremely vigilant about these biases and complete related exposures, individuals in healthcare can sometimes be more likely to suffer health anxiety and overcaution.

Individuals who have these influences in their life tend to have a biased viewpoint on how normal some health-anxious behaviors are. They may not have gotten or may not get accurate feedback about what might be "average" or sufficient health behaviors. They may say something like, "Isn't checking a normal or good thing to do?" The answer to this is that there is no correct answer, only what works best for you as you try to balance your health and your anxiety. If you ask several people, even several experts, you will likely get a great variety of opinions. As we have discussed, most people who are health-anxious are engaging in excessive health behaviors. We encourage you to be mindful of trying to minimize anything you can recognize as likely excessive or unnecessary. However, there will likely be times when you are unsure if your behavior is excessive or not.

As you develop a new way of living that is not based on avoidance of health disasters, we encourage you to consider some long-term approaches to help you decide when to seek appropriate healthcare, and when your behaviors might be likely to hike up anxiety. Below are some guidelines to help you determine what amount of healthcare behaviors may be appropriate for you. Hint: It's likely less than you are doing!

Stop Being Your Own Doctor

There is a reason it takes eight years or more of training to become an MD—because medical practice is complicated! It is not just learning simple rules that can be answered with an internet search, but being taught a complex process of reasoning and inference based on personal experience and knowledge building blocks such as basic chemistry, biology, statistics, and so on. There is a reason why this degree requires experience and many years of practice. So we need to trust that doctors in the medical and psychology fields know more about health practice than us. That being said, of course there are not-so-great doctors out there. We think it is entirely appropriate to try to be generally knowledgeable about your personal health and to practice good preventative health behaviors. This can at times include things like doing some brief(!) research or getting a second opinion. However, asking friends or family, or the internet, for medical information is not a good substitute for your doctor's expertise, and it likely to worsen your anxiety as you encounter more alarming information and try to make sense of conflicting viewpoints.

> Whenever anyone comes in for a cold, especially first-time parents, I always tell them what to look out for. I go through what the warning signs are. I basically tell them to never search anything on Google. I give them guidelines about when to be worried. Like, I say: fever for more than five days, trouble breathing, vomiting profusely, unable to keep down liquids .... I always say, outside of that, if the kid is playful, acting otherwise fine, you don't have to come to the doctor. I give general guidelines. We have an on-call person. You can always call and talk to our triage nurse.
>
> Dr. L., Pediatrician

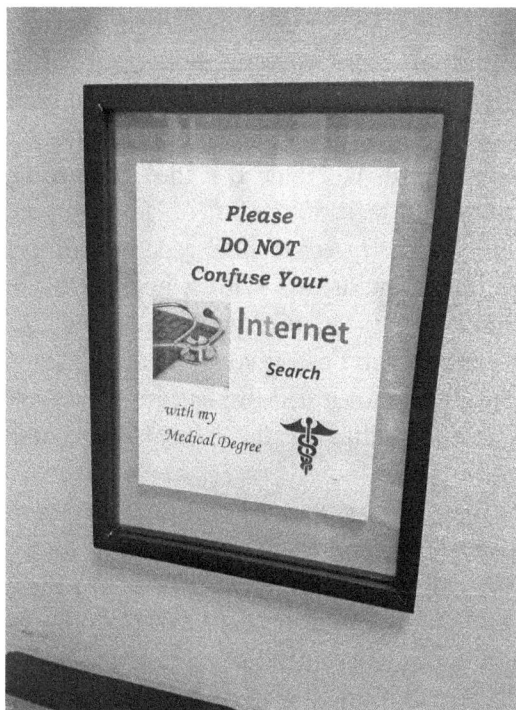

FIGURE 9.1 A tongue-in-cheek sign posted in a doctor's office.

As noted in our section on cyberchondria in Chapter 5, we emphasize limiting internet research about health as much as possible, as it is related to increased illness anxiety in the long-run.

One problem we often encounter in working with individuals with illness anxiety is a sense of overconfidence in their own conclusions and beliefs. They may have had an experience in which a doctor missed something or they felt a medical procedure or course of treatment went badly, and then make an overgeneralized conclusion that they cannot trust medical professionals. They also often are desperate to explain strange symptoms they are noticing that others do not seem to have, which are often maintained by people being over-vigilant to their normal bodily sensations or benign or minor bodily processes or issues. However, this leads people with illness anxiety to be more likely to glom onto fringe theories and stories of rare individuals who had unexplained symptoms that eventually ended in disaster! In doing so, anxious individuals often become more entrenched in their beliefs, and are less likely to integrate evidence that goes against it. For many, it is much more comfortable to have a theory that helps them make sense of things, even if it may be wrong, than to sit with uncertainty and lack of guidance. However, sitting with this uncertainty is exactly what we'd recommend for illness anxiety. Take all your conclusions with a healthy bit of doubt, and act like a scientist would. Could you prove this idea in a court of law? If not, why are you basing your life on it? Given that you have many biases in your thinking because you are anxious, can you outsource your health decisions to a trusted provider?

We also often suggest that people obtain a primary care physician they trust reasonably well, and use that physician as the "gatekeeper" for specialists or additional testing. They are there to triage problems for you. They (or their office) can let you know if you should come in or not, or see a specialist or not, before you do so. They can also tell you what may be signs to look out for if you are concerned about a specific issue. Don't be afraid to ask "How do I know when I should come in?" and follow the guidelines they give you.

When choosing a primary care physician, make sure to seek out one you feel listens to you, does not rush you out the door, and listens to your concerns. Ideally, they will be someone who does not offer a variety of extra tests because they are concerned you will get upset otherwise. Finally, the best doctors are the doctors who know and are willing to say what they do not know, which is often the case. Medicine is often highly educated guesswork, and there are often not clear answers (despite our wanting them!).

Get Appropriate Health Guidance: Use Reputable Scientific Sources, but Not *Too* Scientific!

At times, seeking information is appropriate. We don't want you to be ignorant about health, as that is also not adaptive. We encourage you to be open and honest with your treatment providers if you have concerns or questions, so that they can answer them. We suggest that your providers be your main source of health information.

There are times when seeking additional information may be appropriate. Given that when anxious, people have biases in how they think and tend to overestimate the scariness of outcomes, we have found that sometimes anxious feelings are perpetuated by misinformation or lack of information. At times in treatment, we will intentionally seek health-related data if patients truly feel that they have no sense of how an average human might react in a situation. For example, a person I'm working with may say, "I wash my hands before I eat every single time to avoid getting sick, isn't that what most people do?" Usually, these questions can be answered by looking at your personal experience: What have you done in the past, before you had illness anxiety? What have you seen others around you do? If you truly have no idea and need to get information, make sure that you are getting it from a reputable source. If you already sort of know the answer, your question is likely to be more reassurance-seeking than informative, and seeking additional information will likely backfire to create more anxiety.

Obviously, not all information is created equal! If you must look for information on your own (again, this should be rare), make sure you are using a reputable source. This should be an agency you have heard of that has an excellent scientific reputation, such as the Centers for Disease Control (cdc.gov), National Institutes of Health (nih.gov), or your physician. The National Institutes of Health has an excellent guide online on how to select a reputable medical website for information. We encourage you to visit that document at www.nia.nih.gov/health/how-find-reliable-health -information-online. You can always ask your medical doctor to reach out to their colleagues first, and if they are not able to because of energy or time constraints, you could reach out to the above-mentioned reputable resources. We generally discourage visiting or using the following at all: medical/symptom-related listservs, blogs, or similar online forums. These sites/forums tend to be somewhat focused on rare, minor occurrences, and the self-reporting can be highly biased and distorted. It is easy to get caught up in conspiracy theories, rare cases, or distorted opinions online. We also highly discourage symptom searches, in which you enter in a symptom or set of symptoms you are experiencing to see what it could be a sign of. The search engine will almost always feed you worst-case scenarios! We have found that patients nearly always come away from internet research with more doubt than ever, thinking nearly everything is a sign or symptom of something serious. However, they do not consider that this is often the more rare and unlikely explanation for their symptoms.

As you do this, keep in mind that even experts have biases. People who have specialized expertise or allegiances may have an increased focus on preventing risk in their area. For example, if you ask a police officer if you should ever drive over the speed limit, they will likely say "No way!"—although most drivers do this from time to time and find the risk acceptable when it is only slightly over the speed limit. If you ask an infectious disease expert how much you should wash your hands, they will likely say frequently, every day! Similarly, those in jobs like doctors and nurses who work in emergency rooms, or 911 operators, are repeatedly exposed to the worst-case scenarios day in and day out, which may make it seem like these outcomes are more likely than they really are for the general population. Expertise and knowledge are better than consulting lay sources, but remember that expertise is focused on the person's specific area and likely does not fully consider other factors, like how behaviors factor into anxiety (as they are not anxiety disorder therapists, after all!). It is up to you to weigh the risk and whether you feel it makes sense for you in the long run.

Remember: the more you search for health-related information on the internet, the more the internet will offer to you. Many people are familiar with how artificial intelligence and computer algorithms work, such that health information keeps getting fed to you even when you are not asking for it. Once you search for medical-related issues, these programs will assume you are interested, and more information about health will begin to pop in your social media feeds, advertisements, and query searches.

Over time, this leads to your getting a biased perception of things: it makes health issues seem more likely than they are, because they are popping up everywhere! If you have found that this is already the case for you, we suggest that you go into your search settings every once in a while and deselect any relevant medical/health topics as areas of interest. This will limit how much the programs show you medical information without your directly asking for it. Or, on the opposite end, feel free to start to research fun items (in the opposite direction of your health anxiety), and you will find that more content will start to show up regarding more positive things.

Some patients also choose not to watch or read the news, as they have found the information to be highly biased towards the negative. News reporting tends to be focused on information that will grab attention—therefore, it is more likely to include information about fascinating, rare medical horror stories, and less about boring stories of everyone being healthy with benign symptoms! Higher illness anxiety has been associated with increased exposure to popular media,[1, 2] such as social media and the news. Finally, we also discourage the use of any medical apps or medical-related books unless your doctor has directly recommended them for you.

We also discourage patients from reading medical journals or other overly technical information. Information from scientific medical or health journals is often a respected source of information for professionals, but not a great source of information for the lay public. First, information and statistical information can be very technical, making it more likely that the information is misunderstood. Also, one study in and of itself is often not meaningful—it must be considered along with other findings and replications of similar studies. Typically, these studies and information are meant to be consumed in aggregate by a trained professional who can reconcile the findings with existing information. Too often individuals with illness anxiety read an article or a small set of them and do not seek, read, or encounter other research that may go against this information or disprove the study findings.

Ask a Range of Others Who Do Not Have Health Anxiety

Above, we suggested asking our friends and colleagues to get a general sense of what might be a range of average human behavior for health-related internet use. As we mentioned above, this is a technique we sometimes recommend using if people are truly unsure about what is an average or "normal" amount of health behaviors. Sometimes people come from a family with health anxiety or may have observed several others having serious medical issues, and may have had excessive health behaviors modeled for them. They may say to us that they are unsure what an average person would do.

In treating anxious patients in the office, we will often do a confidential survey of everyone in the office—psychologists, students, administrative staff, and so on, asking a question or two about how often they engage in these behaviors, or when. This doesn't result in giving us a "right" answer, but can give us an idea of a range of what most people might do. As psychologists, we are just two individuals—what we do or believe may be inaccurate as well! We have found that we have learned a lot ourselves in doing this technique!

To give you an illustration, below are two examples of surveys we recently conducted by surveying coworkers and friends. The first patient was concerned that her worry in waiting for a medical test result was abnormal. She reported that she was thinking about the medical test for around an hour each day. We told her that we expected some level of appropriate anxiety while waiting for a medical test, and thought we might personally worry about it for under an hour each day, but were unsure how much others might have this on their mind in a similar situation. We decided to create a confidential survey of the clinic staff with the following question:

If you had to wait for medical testing results (e.g., to see if you or a loved one had cancer), how much do you think you would think about it in an average day?

We ended up getting 16 anonymous responses. Our results are shown in Figure 9.2.

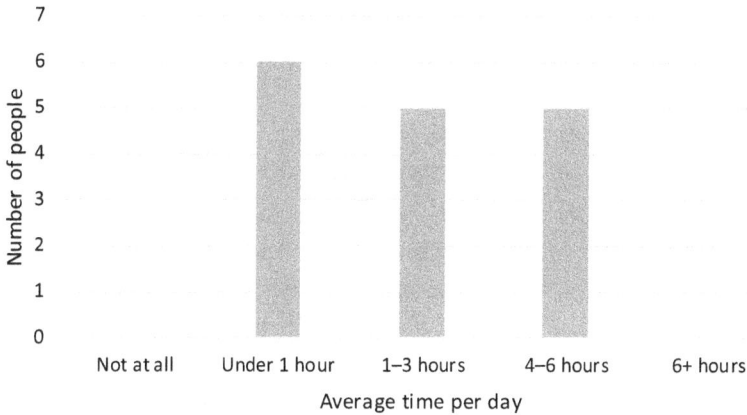

FIGURE 9.2 Survey technique graph

This graph suggests that most people we surveyed reported that in a similar circumstance, they would expect to worry from around zero to six hours per day! No one reported that they wouldn't worry about it at all, and no one reported anticipating more than six hours of worry a day. After discussing the results with the patient, we concluded from this that there is quite a range of how much someone might worry about an important medical test result, and that one hour each day didn't seem all that abnormal, so maybe acceptance of some normal human worry may be a better approach.

If you are unsure about what may be "normal," we encourage you to ask several other people in your life. We obviously suggest that you refrain from asking others who are also excessively anxious about illness. The best people to ask are those you view as competent, trustworthy people who you think will give you an honest answer. However, it is best to get several opinions as this can give you a good range, rather than getting biased opinions from one or two people.

We encourage you to use this sparingly, as we don't want you to obtain excessive reassurance about health. However, we have found that this technique can be very helpful for individuals who think that their health behaviors might be appropriate, but are unsure, or if you feel you truly have no idea about what is a normal frequency of a health behavior. Sometimes people are being quite hard on themselves about behaviors, thoughts, or feelings that are perfectly normal and expected.

However ... Remember That You Have Illness Anxiety, and "Normal" May Not Be Appropriate

Patients of ours often say to us, "Others don't do that, so why should I have to?" This often comes up with regard to exposures. We talked about overlearning exposures in a previous chapter— these are exposures that are designed to really test your fears, and they are often things a typical person might not do on a regular basis, if at all. To really test your fears, we often need to go above and beyond what you encounter ordinarily to be able to teach your brain that things will be OK if you make exceptions to the rules. For example, we are generally taught that washing our hands is a good thing to do after we use the bathroom, and most of us do so without thinking. However, will anything truly bad really happen to us if we don't do wash our hands for a while? We could design an exposure to test this—not wash for several days, maybe, or even touch things in the bathroom such as the toilet seat and not wash after. We have done such things in our clinic many times and found that typically, nothing happens! This can teach our brain that our rules can be more flexible, and that we don't always have to engage in protective behaviors to survive—many of these are done on autopilot.

As exposure therapists, we do a great variety of things that give people pause! For overlearning exposures to treat anxiety disorders, we have done things like eat off shoes, toilets, and public floors, handle cockroaches and snakes, wear silly clothes while shouting, dance in public, make intentional mistakes during work meetings, and ride with patients driving during the worst panic attack of their lives. The point is not to guarantee safety, but to show our brains that some risk is acceptable, and that we often overestimate feared outcomes based on the strength of our feelings. None of these exposures resulted in death or disaster, just the inconvenience of being uncomfortable for a while in different forms. By practicing these things, our distress tolerance muscle (and immune systems!) got stronger.

We encourage you to try to continue to reduce health behaviors and keep them low for as long as possible. For some people, this means never doing them again. While other people may do things like such as watch the news, research medical conditions, and talk with others about medical issues, and so on, you should consider whether these things are working for you in helping you feel less anxious in the long run. Often, they are leading to some short-term relief (which keeps them appealing), but are increasing vigilance and anxiety in the long run. Just like someone who has an addiction to alcohol would be recommended to stay away from bars and friends who drink, we suggest that you stay away from heath behaviors and information if you tend to engage with or seek them excessively.

Like other behavioral issues such as someone who overuses alcohol or someone who is dieting, you may want to restructure things in your environment so that you are not tempted to do these things. This is particularly the case if you tend to engage in many proactive health behaviors (rather than avoid health behaviors). Often this entails several environmental changes to help you stay away from temptation. These can be a variety of things: staying accountable by telling others about your anxiety or plan to reduce health behaviors, talking to friends or family who discuss health with you excessively to let them know that you are trying to not seek reassurance, telling your doctor that you have illness anxiety, limiting how much time you spend on the internet, discontinuing or blocking online health groups, deleting health apps, and so on. The more you can limit temptation, the better. We are unlikely to succeed in tasks that require self-control unless we make many environmental changes in our life, yet many people repeatedly just say, "I will try harder next time." You were already trying hard! Usually, a multifaceted approach is necessary to limit exposure to triggers that tempt you to engage in excessive health behaviors. As you do so, remember to be compassionate with yourself, and remember that you are a work in progress, as we all are, and 100% success is not expected, just your best effort.

Consider Telling Your Doctor That You Have Illness Anxiety

We generally recommend that patients with health anxiety tell their medical providers that they have illness anxiety. We have noticed that some other psychological providers are hesitant to tell patients to do this, as they fear that patients will then not be taken seriously by their doctors, or that doctors will think they are crying wolf. We have rarely found this to be the case; in fact, we have found that doctors have been more patient and willing to hear out patients who have informed them about their health anxiety. In addition, they can be more cautious about what tests they suggest, rather than ordering tests that may not be necessary for you.

There is a lot of overlap between medical conditions and psychological conditions. In fact, we often view psychological conditions as medical issues. There are often a lot of biological influences on anxiety conditions. We believe that your physician can generally treat you better if they are able to factor in your anxiety. They can assess for or rule out biological issues that may explain or contribute to increases in anxiety. They are unable to do this appropriately if they do not know that you are anxious! There is no clear division between mental health symptoms and medical symptoms, and they often overlap. How you think can greatly impact how much you notice and suffer from physical symptoms, and can greatly exacerbate physical symptoms. In turn, this impacts how you behave, which impacts your health, and so on. Everything in this system is linked, and by working on mental health, we can generally improve your overall physical health as well, and vice versa. Keeping these worlds separate limits the ability of your providers to see the whole picture.

It should be noted that many medical providers are not aware that providing excessive reassurance is generally a bad idea for individuals with health anxiety. Therefore, they may often do behaviors that while well-intentioned, backfire for hypochondriacal patients, such as over-explaining things, offering tests to appease, or providing excessive reassurance. You may want to tell them that you are trying to avoid excessive reassurance and overall trying to reduce health behaviors (or, if you are a health behavior avoider, trying to attend appointments regularly and follow recommendations). Alternatively, if you have a psychologist you are seeing for health anxiety, you may want to sign a release of information form which gives them consent to talk to your medical care providers. They may be able to help with explaining that excessive reassurance and help-seeking is back-firing for you.

> *There are a lot of doctors out there that do practice defensive medicine. If a patient complains about something, [the doctor is] always going to order x, y, or z test, even if it's not appropriate. All psych diagnoses in general, I would personally rather know. I always get frustrated working in a facility that has psychiatry involvement because sometimes those psych notes are hidden from us; I will not know the patient has a depression or anxiety diagnosis and what to look out for. I think it would be helpful for doctors to know that someone has health anxiety because I know that the doctor's answer sometimes is to give reassurance, which ends up perpetuating the problem. Not everyone in the medical field is aware that one of the ways that you help [illness anxiety] is to not reassure when you know it's really not a problem, or the thing [the patient is] concerned about is nonexistent, that it's not time for their yearly screening test, and so on.*
>
> *—Dr. L., Internal Medicine*

Draft a Brief List of When to Seek Care

Patients often tell us that they know at this point that their anxious thoughts and health behaviors can be over the top, but that when unexpected physical sensations arise, their anxiety takes over and they impulsively engage in health behaviors. This make sense given our prior discussions of how, when you are anxious, it is often very difficult to make good decisions! Remember that when you are anxious, your attention is biased, such that you pay more attention to information that suggests you are in peril rather than information that things will be OK. Also, much of the worry process is your brain trying to problem-solve what to do—waffling back and forth about issues such as "Should I go to the doctor or not? Is this concern serious enough?" Therefore, you can save time and stress by making some guidelines in advance, while you are in a calmer moment.

If you are someone who tends to seek excessive medical attention or medical advice, we encourage you to draft a short list of types of signs that might help you know when you will decide to seek medical attention, and what level of attention might be appropriate. Obviously, there is no way that you can write down all possible physical sensations you might experience in the future, but we encourage you to focus on some categories that can help you narrow it down, especially focusing on any types of symptoms that may be particularly alarming for you. For example, a patient with a family history of epilepsy was particularly worried any time he noticed any "neurological" signs or symptoms, such as dizziness or difficulty remembering words or names. However, he recognized that he often had these symptoms and that others without medical conditions had them occasionally as well. Therefore, he focused on making a list of which of these types of symptoms might warrant a doctor's visit, and when.

There are no right answers in making this list. Most people have differences of opinion as to when they choose to seek medical attention. In addition, they may seek different types of medical attention. The most important part is that you believe that it is appropriate and helpful for you, that you have some confidence you can follow it, and that you think it will help you decide in the moment about what is appropriate versus excessive medical care.

In writing your list, consider including elements of the following if you think they will help you decide in the moment:

◆ Frequency of symptom
◆ Duration of discomfort
◆ How long you have been experiencing the sensation
◆ Pain level (compared to previous times when you were in pain)
◆ Functional interference (is it stopping you from doing things you want or need to do?)

Other factors to consider when deciding when to seek medical attention or not:

♦ Is there a pattern to the symptoms? That is, do they only occur in specific situations such as when you are in an emotionally stressful situation? Do you not notice them when you are otherwise occupied?

♦ Are the physical symptoms what would be natural and expected as your body ages? Most people experience new and odd symptoms over time, with most of them being benign.

♦ If you had a prior medical issue (e.g., cancer), how similar are your current sensations/symptoms to your previous diagnosis? What have your doctors advised you about how often you should do follow-up and what signs to look out for?

♦ How accurate a reporter are you? When you have thought something was wrong with you in the past, how often were you correct, or did your specific diagnoses emanate from anxiety?

♦ How much time have you given the symptom? Does it resolve on its own? Can you give it a week or two and see if symptoms start to resolve before reaching out for medical assistance?

♦ Are you basing your behavior on the actual here-and-now problem, rather than "what ifs" that haven't happened yet. Is your decision to seek care based on the actual problem in front of you (e.g., an unusual bump/bruise on your wrist that is only slightly painful) or what you think it *could* be (e.g., "Tthis could be/become a pulmonary embolism."). Try to make rules for the problems in front of you, not ones that haven't happened yet!

We encourage you to be very specific in your list. For example, instead of writing "Call a doctor when I have a high fever," write what temperature you are defining as high, how long the fever needs to last before you seek attention, who you will call, and so on.

To provide you with an example, in discussing this with a patient who had tendency to worry about any new symptom that arose, she made a list looking something like the following:

My Medical Decision Chart

Emergency Room or Urgent Care

- ◆ If profusely bleeding and does not stop/clearly need stitches
- ◆ Visible/obvious physical injury (e.g., broken bone), cannot perform a physical action at all (e.g., cannot walk or move a limb)
- ◆ Severe pain (greater than 7/10 pain)

Call My Primary Care Doctor to Make an Appointment as Soon as Possible

- ◆ Pain or discomfort higher than 5/10 for more than 12 hours continuously
- ◆ Blood in stool/urine
- ◆ Continuous or worsening sensations (e.g., dizziness) for more than 24 hours
- ◆ Lump under skin, if hard and not moveable
- ◆ Urinary tract infection (I will know when these happen)
- ◆ Fever over 100° for more than 5 days

Make an Appointment with My Regular Doctor for Follow-up, Not Urgent

- ◆ Continuous symptoms/sensations that last more than 4 days, and/or worsen
- ◆ Pain/discomfort more than 2.5/10
- ◆ Fainting once

Wait and See/Use Over-the-counter Medicine

- ◆ Stomach pain/indigestion
- ◆ Vomiting
- ◆ Back pain, joint pain, or headaches if not continuous or pain is mild
- ◆ Fever over 100° for less than 3 days

Below is a template for you to draft your own list about when you think it is appropriate for you to seek medical attention. Remember to list any signs and symptoms that have been a concern in the past. Also consider what types of symptoms tend to alarm you the most. If new types of sensations or signs arise in the future that concern you, you may want to add them the list if it helps you make decisions in the moment about what level of care may be appropriate for you.

We have found that most people with illness anxiety can do this reasonably well in a calm moment, and at those times tend to show judgment that is like individuals who do not have health anxiety. However, if you feel that your anxiety is still factoring into your decision chart or if you feel truly unsure about when you should seek attention, you may want to ask others you respect (and who do not have health anxiety!) about how they know when to seek medical attention, and what level they seek.

Once you have drafted the list, keep it somewhere easily accessible or visible and follow it when you are noticing a symptom. One patient posted it on her refrigerator so she would not forget it! You may also want to review it regularly to make sure that you remember to follow the guidelines in moments of anxiety.

Sometimes people do not know what types of symptoms may warrant a higher level of care versus a lower one. Some people may use urgent care or the emergency room as their primary care provider, which we do not recommend as it can be costly and time-consuming. To give you some guidelines about what might be a higher versus lower level of care, we spoke with some local emergency rooms and urgent care departments. Again, *this should not be construed as medical advice, and is not a definitive list,* as each case is different. We encourage you to call and ask your medical practice if you are unsure what level of care is recommended. However, we want you to keep in mind that there are several levels of care and urgency.

Urgent care centers (or more rapidly scheduled appointments with a general care provider) generally handle cases such as:

◆ Sprains and fractures
◆ Urinary tract infections

- ◆ Shortness of breath
- ◆ Ear infections
- ◆ Blood in vomit or diarrhea

Emergency rooms tend to be reserved for just that: emergencies! Emergency departments tend to focus on life-threatening issues, commonly dealing with issues such as:

- ◆ Poisonings
- ◆ Electric shock
- ◆ Broken bones
- ◆ Head or spine injuries
- ◆ Severe burns or cuts with uncontrolled bleeding
- ◆ Chest pains or significant difficulty breathing
- ◆ Pregnancy complications
- ◆ Sudden inability to move, speak, or see
- ◆ Seizures

Symptoms that are often considered non-urgent and can probably wait for a scheduled primary care visit (if any medical attention was warranted at all) include:

- ◆ Minor burns
- ◆ Pink eye (conjunctivitis)
- ◆ Sprains
- ◆ Sore throat, potential strep throat, cough
- ◆ Rashes or skin infections
- ◆ Digestive upset, vomiting, or diarrhea
- ◆ Headaches

Remember: everyone is different and may have factors that make their chart look different than others. For example, a person with a significant cardiac history may have been told by their physician to go to the emergency room if they notice any arm pain or chest pain, or someone with years of living with chronic migraines and who expects them may not need to seek a doctor's attention each time one arises. Factor in what you think is appropriate for your health circumstances.

My Medical Decision Chart

<u>Go to emergency room or call ambulance:</u>

<u>Contact my doctor to inquire about an appointment ASAP/go to urgent care:</u>

<u>Schedule a future (not immediate) appointment with my doctor:</u>

<u>Wait and see/do not seek medical attention now:</u>

Now that you have drafted your list to help guide you about what to do when odd, new, and/or uncomfortable symptoms come up, practice with the list of symptoms below. It includes some examples of symptoms that illness-anxious people have fretted about. They had a hard time deciding whether they should seek medical attention, and what level of attention they should seek. Based on your Medical Decision Chart, and keeping in mind that you are trying to refrain from excessive health behaviors as much as possible, what would you do?

Issue	Frequency	Duration	Discomfort/ pain level	What would I do?
Indigestion-like stomach discomfort after eating certain foods, like spicy foods and several fruits.	Each time I eat the food	Has been going on for about a month. Lasts for 30 min to 3 hours.	2/10	
I think I feel a possible small lump in my breast. I had a mammogram 3 months ago that was clear.		I noticed it this week.	0/0	
Dull pain sensation in upper armpit, near top of breast.	Intermittent, maybe once/day	0–15 minutes	2/10	
Notice my heart racing and what feels like heart palpitations, no obvious trigger.	5–30 times/day	Fleeting. Has been going on for about 3 weeks.	1/10	
I feel a tiny (smaller than pencil eraser) soft bump under my skin on my wrist. I worry whether it could be an embolism (blood clot).	Whenever I press the skin in that area	First noticed 3 days ago	0/10	

10

Living a Life in Which Risk and Safety Are Balanced

Check-in on Treatment Homework and Progress

Thought-challenging Practice

If you are still noticing that you are having episodes of strong health anxiety, let's take a step back and check in. Have you been completing the Thought-challenging Form on paper? Most people at this point find that if they have practiced formally writing out their thoughts and challenging them thoroughly, they have noticed some reduction in anxiety. Many people report they are noticing that their brain is beginning to do some thought-challenging automatically. Every time you challenge a thought, you are adding a mental warrior to your army to fight the enemy comprised of all the cognitive distortions you experience. You want to build your army to have a high number of warriors and to become a strong, unbreakable force.

If you have not found a change in your frequency or intensity of anxious thoughts, you may want to take another look at your Thought-challenging Form to make sure you are challenging all the interpretations you are making. Remember that the thought challenging will not take away distress, but it should reduce it, at least a little! If you are finding that you are not noticing any reduction in distress after completing the thought challenging, go back to the drawing board and try to identify what you are really

DOI: 10.4324/9781032711355-10

implying to yourself, and make sure your corrections reflect the literal truth without any distortions. If you are having a hard time doing this on your own, you may want to find a licensed cognitive behavioral therapist to help you identify and challenge thoughts. It seems easy, but identifying what we are implying to ourselves can often be quite hard! Challenging it can be even harder.

Exposure Practice

Let's also check in again as to how you have been doing with the exposures. Have you been doing daily practice of the exposure you selected in Chapter 9? Did you practice that exercise daily for at least a week? Did you refrain from using protective behaviors as much as possible?

Are you avoiding doing the exposures? If you have been avoiding, yet are still feeling motivated to change, you may want to incorporate a schedule for working on these exposures. Can you get someone to help you with follow-through on the exposures? Remember, seeking a trained clinician may be a good idea if you have problem-solved as much as you can and you continue to feel stuck.

If you have been doing the exposure diligently, great job! Step back and look at all the exposures you have done already. You have taken some risks in standing up to the anxiety bully that tells you worst-case scenarios will occur. What have you learned from the exposures you have done so far? How have the exposures been, compared with what you thought they would be like prior to doing them? Have you learned anything about your ability to tolerate distress, and how long it hangs around? How are you thinking about how you have faced your fears—are you giving yourself due credit?

Below is another exposure form to select and track the next exposure you will do next week. Most people do the next exposure on their hierarchy. Usually at this point, people are doing exposure items from the top of their hierarchy. While most people opt to go through their exposures in a gradual way (from lowest to highest level of SUDS), remember: if you are feeling confident that you can shoot higher without using protective behaviors, go for it!

This week's exposure(s):

Anticipated discomfort (SUDS)	My anxious predictions: What do I think will happen when I do this (e.g., will I get hurt, ill, or die)? How uncomfortable will I be, and for how long?	Actual SUDS the final time I did the task this week	Actual outcome

Living a Valued Life and Accepting Anxiety

You cannot be overcautious and unanxious at the same time—what balance will you choose?

Our patients often try to debate with us whether certain health behaviors are appropriate or not. They often try very hard to convince us as clinicians that their choice to engage in the health behavior is rational and appropriate. We try to reorient them that we are not medical doctors—we are not here to tell them which behaviors are appropriate or not! As therapists specializing in anxiety, we can only tell them what is best for treating anxiety. What we know is that in general, the more cautious people are about health, the more anxious they will feel about health. High levels of caution and protective behaviors tend to be related to increased anxiety. The problem is that many hold the belief that they can be very, very cautious regarding health and engage in many health-related behaviors and vigilance, yet simultaneously have the expectation that they should not feel anxious! It is an unrealistic expectation to keep up extreme health vigilance and feel unanxious. The good news is that it is up to you where you would like to set the balance of the scale—how you balance anxious behaviors and caution with making choices that are more

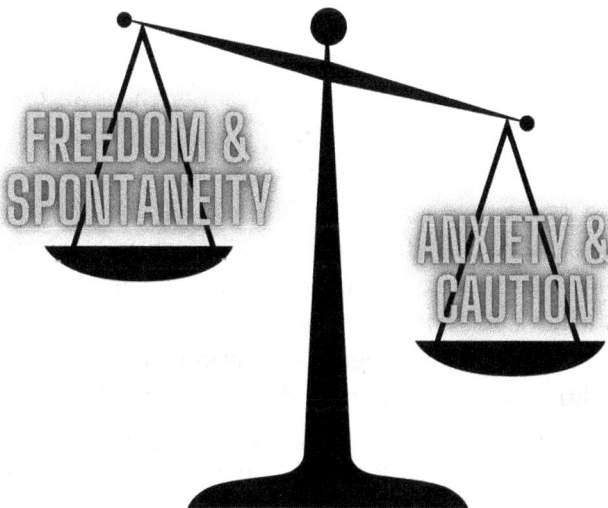

FIGURE 10.1 Scale

likely to lighten your anxiety. Everyone has a different level they set the scale at, based on their own factors, such as motivation, health history, and personal tolerance of anxiety. Some people have personal health as a special priority and are willing to tolerate some anxiety in service of that, so they are somewhat more cautious. Others are on the opposite side and have a stronger value of freedom and spontaneity in life. They may choose to let go of more health behaviors for the sake of enjoying their life with less anxiety. You are free to choose in which direction you would like your scale to tip, and how far.

Accepting the Presence of Distress

We have noticed that many of our patients with illness anxiety have a perfectionistic streak. We do not mean perfectionism in the way that this term can be colloquially used, such as to reflect high cleanliness, meticulousness, or choosiness. We are referencing a commonly used clinical definition, which includes high standards, and frequently a sense that there is usually a correct way to do any given task, and that this correct path must be pursued. Perfectionism also usually carries an exaggerated sense that small mistakes can lead to extremely large consequences.

Because of this perfectionism or otherwise, we often find that patients are harshly judging their own experience of anxiety or distress. They may view it as inappropriate, unusual, pathological, or especially uncomfortable to have or show strong emotions. They may believe that doing so makes them appear flawed to others, that it will interfere with their work or school performance, or that it is otherwise a form of weakness.

Why is this a problem when treating illness anxiety? Research over the past several decades has shown that efforts to block emotions often make them worse in the long run![1, 2] This is something psychologists often call "emotional suppression." This refers to when people try to get rid of negative emotions, fight them off, or otherwise blunt them. This can be done in a variety of ways. Sometimes, the avoidance is obvious to us: trying not to cry, or trying to efface feeling things through use of substances or self-harm behaviors, or not doing things that make us feel intensely anxious. However, as you know by now, avoidance behaviors can also be subtle, such as trying to distract yourself from thinking about something negative, avoiding others when you are feeling anxious, or trying to shut the feelings down and move on. However, as you have learned, avoidance is not generally a great coping technique—it may work well in the short term, but tends to amplify distress in the long run. It also can lead to your experience of the world growing narrower by the day. The more rules you enlist for your own life, the more your life narrows and the more anxious and depressed you can feel.

The difference between those who have problematic anxiety and those who do not is often not the content of the things people worry about, or even how much they worry about it. Research has shown that much of the time, it is how people respond to it. Part of this is how people view their own emotional experience. You can take any bad (or good!) situation and make it especially awful based on how you respond to it. For example, imagine a person with severe chronic pain, or someone who has recently lost a limb. Most people would agree that these are negative events that would distress most people. However, the degree of distress can be greatly impacted by how that person responds to the problem. One individual may choose to focus on the missing limb or pain and ruminate about all the things they can no longer do. They might say all day to themselves "I hate this! Why me? I am so uncomfortable!" They may refrain from doing activities to avoid exacerbating the pain, and instead sit around and not feel miserable. Another individual experiencing the same issue may say, "Well this is a difficult change, but I have decided to cope as best as I can," and try to adapt and pace themself as appropriate. While still distressed, they might have slightly more optimism, and take more initiative do more activities that give them some sense of reward, and that will reduce focus on discomfort and pain in the long run.

In short, if you tell yourself that anxiety is awful to have, it will most definitely will be. The good news is that you have some control over how you appraise your anxiety experience. In addition, your ability to tolerate anxiety can likely improve with practice, as you have hopefully learned by now from exposure experience! This is something the psychology field often refers to as "distress tolerance"—or your ability to tolerate negative emotions like anxiety, depression, sadness, and grief. To tolerate these emotions is to continue to do what is most important to you without excessively trying to suppress or fight off negative emotions, and accepting that they are part of the human experience. Research has shown that people who have higher distress tolerance are more likely to have better mental health outcomes in a variety of areas, including (but not limited to) less suicidality, impulsivity, substance abuse, depression, and anxiety, and better general perceived quality of life.[3-7] The good news is that some research studies examining how to increase distress tolerance have suggested that it is likely a skill you can develop with practice, and that practicing exposures may help increase your distress tolerance.[8-11]

You do not need to fight off any emotion, and it's OK to have anxiety or distress. What is often so interfering for people is the way they respond to it. If you avoid and catastrophize, you will have interference and distress. This may sound like a lot of responsibility, but it is actually freeing—you have some control of how you respond to your anxiety! Related to this, it's OK to experience other feelings that come along with health anxiety, such as grief, sadness, and anger. So many times, patients are trying to not feel sad about the potential of dying and being separated from their family—we would expect you to be sad about this, and would be more concerned if you did not feel sad in thinking about it! That feeling of sadness in this instance tells us that your family is an important value to you. The most important things in life come along with great distress, not a lack of distress. Take a moment now and think about the most meaningful times in your life. Did great highs come along with some distress? Most people say that in the most powerful moments in their lives, during things such as births, graduations, and accomplishments, they had great joy, but that there was also significant distress in the process. Living a valued life means allowing yourself to take this risk of feeling these things. Sometimes, with great pleasure comes great discomfort. They do not have to be mutually exclusive.

There are many good books, online guides, videos, and therapists out there who are trained in how to increase distress tolerance. Many cognitive behavioral-type psychological treatments (that you may have heard of) have elements of specific components that are designed to increase a person's distress tolerance. These treatments have been proven to be helpful in reducing a great variety of distress in many mental health areas such as depression, anxiety, personality disorders, substance use disorders, chronic pain, and so on. If you think this applies to you, or you are interested in such a treatment, you may want to look up a therapist (or book or online materials) whot discusses what is known as acceptance and commitment therapy (ACT). You may have also heard the term "mindfulness." Mindfulness is a meditation practice often used in the context of ACT to aid in increasing a person's distress tolerance by getting some distance between them and their thoughts. However, we should remind you that the goal of these approaches is not to remove anxiety, but rather to accept that it is there sometimes, and to learn to coexist with it. We talk about this a little more below.

Living According to Your Values, Not Your Anxiety

At this point, we hope that your anxiety has substantially reduced, but it is likely that it is not gone, and will require ongoing practice for quite a while. You may feel hard on yourself that you have not accomplished what you want, or that you just aren't as free of anxiety as you may have been in the past.

It's important to have realistic expectations, so let's make sure we talk about that here: lapses in skills are expected, and we do not expect perfection from you! In fact, expectation for perfection is what causes a great deal for anxiety. Instead, step back and think about whether you are working towards the goals you have for reducing anxiety, or if modifications to your plan need to be made. We can often tell that some patients are crossing their fingers hoping they will magically go back to a time when they seemingly were low in anxiety and did not have the anxious voice bullying them at every turn. However, this treatment is meant to give a new and improved version of yourself, not return you a place you were previously in your life. Rather than being a source of avoidance and distress, anxiety can be a catalyst for great growth.

As we mentioned above, people can tolerate a great deal of distress if that distress is experienced on the journey of working towards goals that are important to them. Having to do something anxiety-provoking simply because you are telling yourself you *should* often feels more painful than doing it because it lies on the path to something you value in your heart. For example, studying long hours in the evenings is not fun for most people, but may feel less bad if you are dreaming about becoming an emergency medical technician; mothers endure painful childbirth as they are anticipating the joy of a child, and so on. As we discussed above, distress often comes at times along with great joys in life. Now that you have begun to face your anxiety bully to stop living a life in avoidance of distress, let's talk about what you *want* from life. Many people don't know their mission statement for their life. Sometimes, people have been living in an avoidance-based style for so long they have not even thought about what they would seek in life that would be fulfilling. So let's think a bit about what you want from life, discomfort or not. Certainly, it isn't to avoid feeling anxious at all costs.

Take some time to think about what your most important values are and fill out the blanks below. Before you do, here are some notes. First, we mention the word "values" quite often. We define values as broad constructs that someone might aspire to: things such as honesty, feeling spiritually connected, being present for friends when needed, educating others, being a good role model for one's children, and so on. Values are so broad that we never fully achieve them, as there is always more that can be done to work on a value. A value should be something you desire, rather than something you are trying to avoid. It should also be something you truly want, rather than something you *think you should* want. Many people with anxiety are so oriented towards doing things right that they tell we clinicians what they think we want to hear, or write down what they think are "correct" answers, rather than what would really motivate them.

What are your top values?

_____

_____

_____

_____

If you are feeling stuck, below are some commonly cited values to get you brainstorming (although don't feel that you have to choose any of these).

Kindness to animals	Cultural tradition	Closeness with friends
Giving back	Sense of humor	Financial stability
Spending time with family	Empathy for others	Sharing my skills
Job competence	Enjoying nature	New experiences/curiosity
Education/growth	Independence	
Perseverance	Creative self-expression	

Now that you have identified some of your top values, which do you think might be your top three values? If they directly came into conflict with each other, which might you choose? (Remember they are not set in stone, and you can change your mind about your top values at any time.)

Top values:

1) _____

2) _____

3) _____

Now take a close look at your life and your daily actions. Do you think you are living in service of these top values, or are you living a life based on trying to get away from anxiety?

_____

_____

_____

_____

How is your illness anxiety continuing to prevent you from working towards these values? How has that contributed to how you feel? How would you be behaving differently if you were working towards your values, rather than trying to avoid anxiety?

_____

_____

_____

_____

Positive Preventative Health Behaviors and Adaptive Forms of Avoidance

By now you know that coping strategies such as avoidance, rumination, and overprotection tend to create increased levels of anxiety. Behaviors that are associated with less anxiety and an increased sense of mental well-being include appropriate planning for problems, less engagement in rumination, accurate self-talk and more optimistic interpretations, and more acceptance of emotional experiences.[12-15]

Good self-care is one of the most important ways to appropriately reduce health risk and overall stress and anxiety. However, many people react intensely to intermittent symptoms, rather than simply trying to engage in health-protective behaviors in advance.

Self-care to reduce stress and anxiety involves things like a healthy diet, good sleep hygiene, exercise, socializing with others, and good work–life balance. People tend to underestimate the impact these things have on their daily stress levels and overall health! It is very difficult to reduce stress and anxiety if you do not have a decent self-care foundation and are not sleeping, are active, engaging in too many activities, and so on. Some of the best health behaviors are proactive rather than reactive.

How are you being proactive in reducing stress by regularly engaging in health behaviors (such as doctor's check-ups as prescribed, healthy eating, exercise, sleep hygiene, engagement with social contacts)? Are you lacking in any of these areas?

_____

_____

_____

_____

If you are lacking in any of the self-care areas, no need to worry—these behaviors can hard to keep up with, especially if you are not in the habit of doing them. Often people are setting goals too high and end up not doing anything because the goal was too difficult! Are there small but doable ways that you can begin to work towards better self-care in your daily life? For example, can you walk the dog a little bit longer? Try a more regular sleep and/or wake time? Reduce some responsibilities if you are feeling overwhelmed? Meet with more friends in person to increase your support from others (and build a healthy immune system with appropriate exposure to germs)?

Small areas I may be able to practice better self-care to proactively make myself more resilient to anxiety and stress episodes:

_____

_____

_____

_____

246 ◆ Balancing Risk and Safety

Also, while we have thoroughly discouraged you from avoiding things that make you anxious, there are some times that avoidance can be adaptive. We recommend approaching anxious situations if they are things that you want or need to do, or are getting in the way of your daily life. However, there are many situations that people expose themselves to that increase anxiety that are unnecessary! For example, many patients decide to reduce or stop talking about health with others when possible, avoid or reduce watching or reading the news or using social media platforms and so on. These activities are things people often feel compelled to do, but tend to be triggers for increased anxiety, and are optional. If you are engaging in such activities, take a close look at the function these behaviors are serving for you. Are you engaging in them to prevent anxiety (e.g., because you might miss out on some important health information), or because you feel you *should*--or are they truly making your life more fulfilling?

Ways I might begin to avoid unnecessary exposure to health cues (limiting how much you talk about health with others, limiting talking about health with others, limiting exposure to health-related information on social media, etc.)?

_____

_____

_____

_____

Hopefully by now you are having less daily anxiety related to health. However, you may remain concerned about symptoms flaring back up when you a sudden new or unusual bodily sensation or problem arises. When those times arise, anxiety may escalate quickly, and therefore the anxiety voice may try to take over directing you right away. Anxiety builds neuronal based networks in our brain that become reactivated when we encounter a similar feeling, situation, experience, or person. When people complete successful exposure-based treatment, we do see this response become more like non-anxious brains, but the old ways of thinking do not disappear entirely. It is important in those moments that you recognize the anxiety is not suddenly back in full force, but that it is conditioned to reappear and you have the behavioral (exposure) and cognitive (thought-challenge) skills to combat your anxiety.

Your insight into the anxiety voice may not be fully strong yet, so we encourage you to write a bit of a reminder to yourself. Now that you are in a colder moment, what would you tell the version of you that tends to get overanxious about health signs? Based on what you have learned, what would you say to that version of you, if you could meet them face-to-face in an anxious moment? Also imagine and respond to the skepticism that you know you might express when you are anxious. How might you respond to anxious thoughts such as "I have been fine before, but now could be the time something really disastrous is happening!" or "how do I know if I should see the doctor or not?"

Remember that you view all incoming information through certain filters. Sometimes these will be your old filter (and it is important you recognize that) and sometimes it will be your new and improved filter. It is important to recognize that your filter may not always be an accurate representation of reality or your risk of getting or having an illness. Be your own skeptic and question your thoughts and motives when it comes to anxiety around medical issues. Instead of preventing future medical issues, try and embrace them. Having to experience the changes that come with age, mean that you have been given the chance to get older. Lots of people get to be young, but not everyone gets the opportunity to grow older.

11

Moving Forward and Embracing a Full Life

Your Love–hate Relationship with Anxiety

While you may think your anxiety is uncomfortable and that you unequivocally want it to go away, usually our relationship with anxiety is a love–hate one. Even when certain actions or ways of thinking cause us great discomfort, we often persist with them because they are rewarding in other ways. For example, we may have the feeling that if we worry enough in advance, somehow it will lead to less disappointment in the future. Or we may feel less guilt that we are not taking care of our health in more concrete ways (e.g., eating right and exercising). Or we may just find it comfortable because it is a predictable, familiar way of thinking, even if it is negative! Even when we are very negative and anxious, sometimes those behaviors are serving a purpose for us, or at least we *think* they are. Psychologists sometimes refer to this as an "ego-syntonic" relationship. Ego-syntonic means that there is a part or the entire whole of you that believes the anxiety you feel about your health works for you. That is, you believe the anxious voice, believe it has a protective value, and you want to hold onto it as something you value. There may have been legitimate times when your health/illness anxiety prevented you from getting seriously ill or helped you heal faster. This can be very reinforcing for your anxiety. There may be times when your anxiety did help,

DOI: 10.4324/9781032711355-11

but it is not as many as you may think it is. Because of biases in thinking, we are more likely to remember times when those protective behaviors saved us from medical disaster, and discount all the times when anxiety backfired or sucked joy out of our lives.

On the other side of the love–hate coin is the "hate" aspect, or what we would technically term ego-dystonic. Ego-dystonic means that the anxiety you feel is in opposition to your core values and is something you want to leave or eliminate from your life immediately. Sometimes this can feel like a bully who stands beside you and says awful things to try to get you riled up. You may know that the bully is incorrect, but it is still awful to have them there prodding you! You can feel a sense of urgency, disgust, and all-around dislike of what you are experiencing, so much so that it makes you very motivated to get rid of it. It can help if you recognize that this anxiety is a bully who tries to provoke you, but is no more than that: it is just a voice, it is not *you*. Even if a bully is trying to persuade you otherwise, you can still choose how you want to behave. As psychologists, we find the ego-dystonic perspective really helps to fuel and motivate you to stick with your plan to fight against your health/illness anxiety. Unfortunately, patients with illness anxiety often find themselves in the camp of ego-syntonic rather than ego-dystonic. We tell you this to increase your awareness, so that you can step back and decide whether your anxious thoughts and behaviors are really how you want to live your life.

Relatedly, think of what function the anxiety may be serving for you, or at least how you think it is helping you. Is it working in the intended way over the long term? For example, if it is to help you feel fewer negative emotions in the long run, have you found that to be the case? We would also like you to think about the times in your life when your health anxiety led to a productive result rather than just more worry and anxiety. Can you think of these times? Sometimes your brain will say, "See if it worked there, I should be worrying all the time because it helped me in this one particular case." While that may be true, we want to help your brain differentiate the times when your anxiety led to a helpful, productive result versus when it just led to more health anxiety.

What is your relationship with your health anxiety? After going through the workbook, we hope that we have moved you forward to place most of your health anxiety in the ego-dystonic category. Yet we also recognize that it's been your long-time companion now, and as much as you may dislike it, there are parts of you that want to keep it around.

If I Am Not Living with My Health Anxiety, What Will I Spend My Time On?

We often hear, "I've spent so much time on my anxiety, how am I supposed to just give it up? I'm not sure what else to do with my time and myself, as I have spent so long getting used to worrying all the time." Does this sound familiar to you?

For those who do have health anxiety, a significant portion of their day may have been spent on managing the anxiety, such as trying to determine how to avoid the anxiety and how to justify and explain it away to ourselves and others. However, if the goal of our workbook is to reduce your health anxiety over the long run, we need to address what will happen to the copious amounts of time you have previously devoted to it. We must now think of how will we replace the time and effort you have already been putting into anxiety into ways that prevent it from creeping back into your life over the long term.

Although health-related anxiety is the enemy you have been working on combatting, in some ways we can feel a void when it decreases. Sometimes we find that there is a conflictual relationship we can have with our anxiety. Sometimes dealing with empty time and space in our lives can cause a significant amount of anxiety in and of itself, and can lead us to feel the temptation to occupy that space with old, anxiety-increasing habits.

Look back on your week, and see how much of your week is spent worrying or focusing on the anxiety caused by your health anxiety. While we will assume it has improved since you began this workbook, you may still have episodes of time devoted to thinking about your anxiety. It may even be helpful to think of how much time you spent on your illness/health anxiety at the beginning of this workbook compared to where you are now. That way, you can achieve a current assessment of your risks (to fall back into old patterns of illness anxiety) and also see how far you have come. It is possible to lose momentum on the implementation of your skills and have some anxiety creep back in (sometimes more than others), but your mind will not be erased of all the tools and skills you have learned. That is some pretty great news!

Use the following template below to track how you spend your time (remember you can also complete this assessment for where you think you were at the start of this workbook for a comparison).

Time management planner

TIME	ACTIVITY (WORK, ANXIETY THOUGHTS, EXERCISE, ETC)	NOTES

FIGURE 11.1 Time management planner

Think back to when we talked about accepting some distress and living a full life. We discussed how you can plan out your life and achieve your goals and not have them dependent on the limits of anxiety. Anxiety can close your world in and close you off from the world, so it is important to open your world back up and plan to live in it without the influence of anxiety. How does that feel? What do you think of a world and a life you are living where your anxiety does not dictate decisions for you?

Think about how your time has been divided up. How did you spend your time at the beginning of this workbook? How are you currently spending your time? Most importantly, how would you like to spend your time in the future?

Not that you have thought about how you allocate your time, we recommend starting to work on a goals and prioritization list. What have your health worries taken away from you? Are you spending less time on a romantic relationship or interests? Have you found the right place and location to live? What does your social life look like? What does your work life look like? A lot of times, your interests will suffer because of your health anxiety. Some of our patients will spend their entire day at their job, come home, eat, do chores, and with the little free time they have, dedicate that to their health anxiety. As you can imagine, it leads to an exhausting life in service of avoiding discomfort, with little or no pleasure.

Think of what you have lost or not pursued because of your health/illness anxiety. If you ask yourself the question, "What do I miss doing (e.g., hobbies)?" and if you cannot find an answer or you say none, the answer is likely a resounding "yes" that your health/anxiety has driven your decisions for so long that you can no longer even identify what your potential interests are. Think back to times in your life when you felt exhilarated or energized by an activity. We do not have to reinvent your wheel here, just think about activities that used to make you feel engaged, and that can be the place to start! Are there any trips that you have not been on? Any places you would like to go to? We want to encourage you to think of a new "bucket list" for the next six months to a year to regain in your life what your health anxiety has taken from you.

Please take some time to fill out the following list (Figure 11.2). You can even ask friends and family what they think your health/anxiety has taken from your life or their relationship with you.

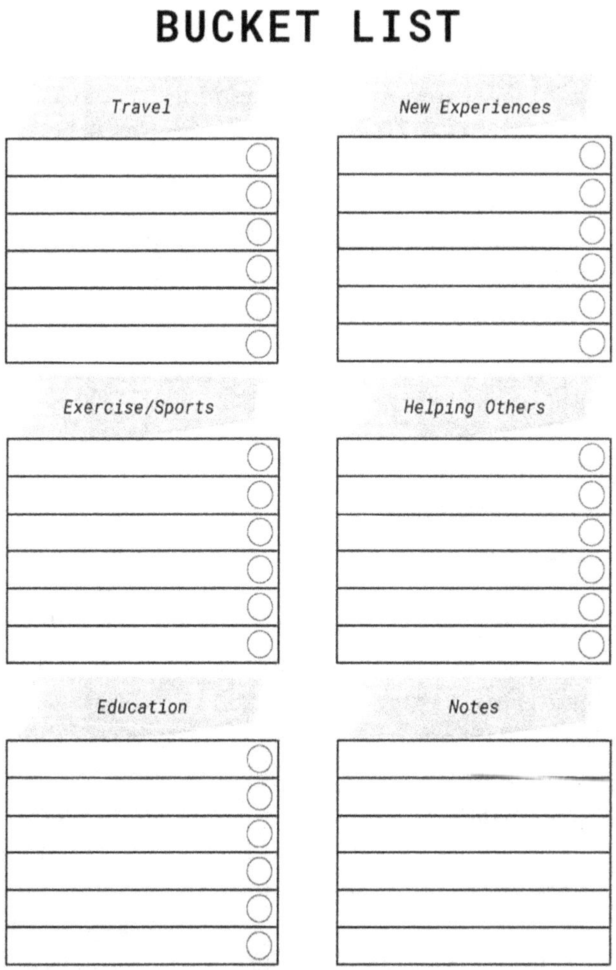

BUCKET LIST

Travel

New Experiences

Exercise/Sports

Helping Others

Education

Notes

FIGURE 11.2 Bucket list

In doing this, some of you may recognize that you are doing the activities and engagements you would like, but your mind still spends a great deal of time worrying during them. These worries occupy your thoughts and distract you from being in the moment. We recommend you continue challenging your thoughts and engaging in exposure before an event. Also, your reaction to your excessive worry is a large part of what keeps it going, and keeps it feeling so keen. Remember that as you practice doing what you want, without safety behaviors, this worry should reduce over time, but until it is practiced quite a bit, anxiety will come along for the ride. If you believe worry is not helpful, practice gently redirecting your attention to the activities and sensory experiences in front of you. Practice listening to what others say, and observe yourself, them, and your situation without any judgment. Allow your anxiety to be present, but temporarily be moved to the corner. This will allow you the mental space to fully engage and be present in the moment.

Relapse Prevention

As you make the transition from spending your effort, energy, thoughts, feelings, and actions on your health anxiety, you will inevitably feel the pull to go back to your old anxious thoughts and habits. You might not even notice that it is happening. It can feel very natural to get pulled back into an anxious style of thinking. Even if you are feeling much better with your illness anxiety, we recommend continuing to practice skills for at least the first three months after you complete this workbook. What does that mean? Well, it means checking in with your workbook and reminding yourself of your skills at least twice per week.

Unfortunately, many of our patients with health anxiety leave treatment before they get to the relapse prevention stage, arguably the most important stage of treatment. Not engaging in a relapse prevention plan and practicing that plan usually means we are more likely see a patient back in our office in the future. Engaging in relapse prevention skills can give you years of not having to re-enter treatment, if not a lifetime.

Remember, the term "relapse" does not mean that you relapse or return to where you were at the beginning or outset of treatment. What it means is that there has been a significant slide back into old anxiety habits, such as looking up information on the internet or repeatedly seeking the medical opinions of doctors because you are feeling anxious (and not due what we have defined as more legitimate symptoms). You can expect a certain amount of backsliding when it comes to your health/illness anxiety, especially during times when health problems flare up, but it is important for you to keep a watchful eye. It is very important to be fully honest and raw with yourself about where you are in your treatment before moving on to the following steps.

Re-assessment of Your Symptoms

A common practice in cognitive behavioral therapy is to measure and intermittently reassess what we are working on. We do this to make sure that we are reaching our goals, and to assess whether what we are doing is helping us reach our goals. Change in anxiety tends to happen gradually, and we might not remember how anxious we were when we started!

Now is a good time to re-take the illness anxiety questionnaire you completed at the beginning of the book. We include it below so that you can re-complete it. You can compare your score to the score you had at the beginning of this book. Did your score improve (lower)? What areas still need to be worked on? If you have been doing the exposures daily, you should be noticing some improvement in your anxiety.

Health Anxiety Inventory (Short Version)[1]

Each question in this section consists of four statements. Please read each group of statements carefully, then select the one which best describes your feelings, over the past six months. Identify the statement by circling the letter next to it—i.e. if you think that statement (a) is correct, circle statement (a); it may be that more than one statement applies, in which case, please circle any that are applicable.

1. (a) I do not worry about my health
   (b) I occasionally worry about my health
   (c) I spend much of my time worrying about my health
   (d) I spend most of my time worrying about my health

2. (a) I notice aches/pains less than most other people (of my age)
   (b) I notice aches/pains as much as most other people (of my age)
   (c) I notice aches/pains more than most other people (of my age)
   (d) I am aware of aches/pains in my body all the time

3. (a) As a rule I am not aware of bodily sensations or changes
   (b) Sometimes I am aware of bodily sensations or changes
   (c) I am often aware of bodily sensations or changes
   (d) I am constantly aware of bodily sensations or changes

4. (a) Resisting thoughts of illness is never a problem
   (b) Most of the time I can resist thoughts of illness
   (c) I try to resist thoughts of illness but am often unable to do so
   (d) Thoughts of illness are so strong that I no longer even try to resist them

5. (a) As a rule I am not afraid that I have a serious illness
   (b) I am sometimes afraid that I have a serious illness
   (c) I am often afraid that I have a serious illness
   (d) I am always afraid that I have a serious illness

6. (a) I do not have images (mental pictures) of myself being ill
   (b) I occasionally have images of myself being ill
   (c) I frequently have images of myself being ill
   (d) I constantly have images of myself being ill

7. (a) I do not have any difficulty taking my mind off thoughts about my health
   (b) I sometimes have difficulty taking my mind off thoughts about my health
   (c) I often have difficulty in taking my mind off thoughts about my health
   (d) Nothing can take my mind off thoughts about my health

8. (a) I am lastingly relieved if my doctor tells me there is nothing wrong
   (b) I am initially relieved but the worries sometimes return later
   (c) I am initially relieved but the worries always return later
   (d) I am not relieved if my doctor tells me there is nothing wrong

9. (a) If I hear about an illness I never think I have it myself
   (b) If I hear about an illness I sometimes think I have it myself
   (c) If I hear about an illness I often think I have it myself
   (d) If I hear about an illness I always think I have it myself

10. (a) If I have a bodily sensation or change I rarely wonder what it means
    (b) If I have a bodily sensation or change I often wonder what it means
    (c) If I have a bodily sensation or change I always wonder what it means
    (d) If I have a bodily sensation or change I must know what it means

11. (a) I usually feel at very low risk for developing a serious illness
    (b) I usually feel at fairly low risk for developing a serious illness
    (c) I usually feel at moderate risk for developing a serious illness
    (d) I usually feel at high risk for developing a serious illness

12. (a) I never think I have a serious illness
    (b) I sometimes think I have a serious illness
    (c) I often think I have a serious illness
    (d) I usually think that I am seriously ill

13. (a) If I notice an unexplained bodily sensation I don't find it difficult to think about other things
    (b) If I notice an unexplained bodily sensation I sometimes find it difficult to think about other things
    (c) If I notice an unexplained bodily sensation I often find it difficult to think about other things
    (d) If I notice an unexplained bodily sensation I always find it difficult to think about other things

14. (a) My family/friends would say I do not worry enough about my health
    (b) My family/friends would say I have a normal attitude towards my health
    (c) My family/friends would say I worry too much about my health
    (d) My family/friends would say I am a hypochondriac

For the following questions, please think about what it would be like if you had a serious illness of a type which particularly concerns you (such as heart disease, cancer, multiple sclerosis, and so on). Obviously, you cannot know for definite what it would be like; please give your best estimate of what you *think* might happen, basing your estimate on what you know about yourself and serious illness in general.

15. (a) If I had a serious illness I would still be able to enjoy things in my life quite a lot
    (b) If I had a serious illness I would still be able to enjoy things in my life a little
    (c) If I had a serious illness I would be almost completely unable to enjoy things in my life
    (d) If I had a serious illness I would be completely unable to enjoy my life at all

16. (a) If I developed a serious illness there is a good chance that modern medicine would be able to cure me
    (b) If I developed a serious illness there is a moderate chance that modern medicine would be able to cure me
    (c) If I developed a serious illness there is a very small chance that modern medicine would be able to cure me
    (d) If I developed a serious illness there is no chance that modern medicine would be able to cure me

17. (a) A serious illness would ruin some aspects of my life
    (b) A serious illness would ruin many aspects of my life
    (c) A serious illness would ruin almost every aspect of my life
    (d) A serious illness would ruin every aspect of my life

18. (a) If I had a serious illness I would not feel that I had lost my dignity
    (b) If I had a serious illness I would feel that I had lost a little of my dignity
    (c) If I had a serious illness I would feel that I had lost quite a lot of my dignity
    (d) If I had a serious illness I would feel that I had totally lost my dignity

---

To remind you, each item on the questionnaire is scored on a scale of 0–3 (i.e., a = 0, b = 1, c = 2, d = 3). Based on your score, how much have you declined on this scale from when you completed it at the beginning of the workbook in Chapter 17? In doing illness anxiety treatment in the clinic, we aim for a change of at least six points on this scale. We call this level of change "reliable change," which just is a statistical way of saying that if someone has shown this decrease, they have shown a decrease that is unlikely to happen just by chance. If your score has reduced, congratulations! Keep up the good work! If your score has not changed, or worsened, you may want to consider reaching out to an anxiety treatment provider who can walk you through the skills or assess what barriers there might be to completing the practice in this book or to benefitting from it. We talk more about this below.

We recommend making a very specific plan about how often you will practice skills from this book, and how much, for the next few months at least. Even if you are feeling better, remember that illness anxiety tends to go up and down, and can flare up at times when you are having strange physical symptoms (which will definitely happen in the future!). Therefore, it's best to practice ahead of time and be ready to reduce the impact of anxiety, rather than waiting for it to hit you.

We encourage you to make a written plan. Usually, these plans involve tapering off the practice you are doing as it gets easier for you. For example, let's say that you are currently doing exposure exercises four times a week for 30 minutes each, and challenging your thoughts every day when anxious thoughts arise. We might recommend the following.

Step 1 (Exposures on the Calendar Below)
For two weeks, do exposures two or three times per week for 30 minutes each (you can choose which days, but we would recommend spacing them apart (e.g., Monday, Wednesday, Friday), and continuing to challenge your thoughts every day. See the example calendar in Figure 11.3.

Step 2 (Exposures on the Calendar Below)
Following step 1, do exposure twice each week for 20 minutes each. Continue to challenge your thoughts every day.

Step 3 (Exposures on the Calendar Below)
Once-weekly exposures and continuing to challenge your thoughts every day. You may want to move into once- or twice-a-month exposures.

From the sample practice plan above, you may be able to see that your active involvement in effortful skill practice tends to decrease over time as symptoms decline, but does not stop altogether. While exposure therapy is an active ingredient of treatment and during the active phase of treatment, it should be used purposefully and judiciously during relapse prevention.

Remember that these are just rough guidelines, so will do not fit everyone. If your illness anxiety begins to rise back up, you may want to increase the frequency of exposures and cognitive challenging that you do, and review the materials from the beginning of the book. It is important to engage in a relapse prevention program, as described above, However, it is also important to recognize that even after your relapse prevention program is done, you may have a spike in your symptoms. This means you may need to go back to being more involved in your previous treatment program (i.e., the first month of relapse prevention). As evidence-based clinicians, we place a lot of emphasis and

SUN	MON	TUE	WED	THU	FRI	SAT
	1 END OF TREATMENT	2	3 EXPOSURE	4	5 EXPOSURE	6
7 EXPOSURE	8	9 EXPOSURE	10	11 EXPOSURE	12	13 EXPOSURE
14	15 EXPOSURE	16	17 EXPOSURE	18	19 EXPOSURE	20
21	22 EXPOSURE	23	24	25 EXPOSURE	26	27
28	29 EXPOSURE	30	31 EXPOSURE			

JANUARY

FIGURE 11.3 Exposure planning calendar, month 1

SUN	MON	TUE	WED	THU	FRI	SAT
				1	2	3
4	5 EXPOSURE	6	7	8 EXPOSURE	9	10
11	12	13 EXPOSURE	14	15	16 EXPOSURE	17
18	19	20 EXPOSURE	21	22	23 EXPOSURE	24
25	26	27 EXPOSURE	28	29		

FEBRUARY

FIGURE 11.4 Exposure planning calendar, month 2

MARCH

SUN	MON	TUE	WED	THU	FRI	SAT
					1	2
3	4	5 EXPOSURE	6	7	8	9
10	11	12	13	14	15	16
17	18	19	20	21	22	23
24	25	26	27	28	29	30
31						

FIGURE 11.5 Exposure planning calendar, month 3

importance on not struggling on your own for too long before seeking out a professional.

If you have been practicing the skills in the book, it is likely that you have come a long way, although likely your health-related anxiety is not *gone*. Continued practice will help keep it reducing over time. You may even feel that you are doing well now. However, in those times when problems flare up, insight often goes out the window a bit (or a lot). As you know by now, when we are anxious, we do not think entirely clearly. Therefore, catching anxiety early in the cycle can make it so that we can see it and begin to implement the strategies we know to reduce it.

Now that you are having less anxiety, the last task we recommend that you do is write a letter to yourself: the version of you that started this workbook. Now that you are in a calmer moment, If you could stand next to the version of you that is or was in peak panic over health, what would you tell them? What would you suggest that they do? How would you address their "yes, but" rebuttals? How would you be supportive and kind to them? What would you tell them about what you have learned from this treatment? On the next page, really take some time to write yourself a compassionate letter that reminds you of what you know, what do to, and how far you have come.

From: Me
To: Anxious Me

Knowing yourself, write a letter to the version of you when you were most anxious about health, if you could meet them face-to-face. What do you know now that might be helpful?

_____

_____

_____

_____

_____

_____

_____

_____

_____

_____

_____

_____

_____

_____

Now that you have written your letter carefully, you may want to include re-reading it in your relapse plan. How often will you review the letter, and when—weekly? When you start to notice weird symptoms? How will you remember to review it?

Reaching Out to a Professional

We recommend that if you are continuing to feel anxious about your health, or if you are getting better at a slower rate than you desire, it may be time to reach out for extra professional support. Remember that illness anxiety is common, and seeking professional support is common, and there are many reasons people do so. For example, our personal viewpoint or perspective can be limited when it comes to having insight about ourselves and our anxious behaviors. An outside point of view can be helpful. Sometimes it also helps to have someone to be accountable to, as designing exposures and trying to do them on your own can be difficult. It can be easy to procrastinate!

We won't sugarcoat it: finding the right therapist can be tricky. There are factors like payment/insurance, finding someone who is knowledgeable about CBT for illness anxiety, and finding someone who is currently taking new patients. As not all therapists do CBT or specialize in the same types of treatments and diagnoses, it is OK to spend 10–15 minutes each talking to a number of different therapists to get a sense of what they offer. We encourage you to tell them what is important in a therapeutic relationship to you. For example, you may want someone who is open, honest, and straightforward, or you may want someone who is more gentle and slower-paced. While we recognize it may not be easy at times, we encourage you to be honest with your provider about what you are looking for, as that will make more a more positive experience with your treatment provider and help them address your concerns rather than trying to mind-read! Feeling comfortable with your therapist—such as feeling like your therapist listens to you and that you agree on what you are both working on—is a significant factor in how much people stick with treatment and how much they benefit from it.[2, 3]

Although we identified the therapeutic relationship as most important in terms of whether you have a positive result from treatment, for illness/health anxiety it is particularly important to receive the right type of treatment. We would recommend seeking out an evidence-based clinician. Unfortunately, we have encountered many clinicians who claim to do CBT but do not adhere to a CBT methodology. Therefore, assessing the quality of CBT can be difficult, but if we have to make one recommendation, it would be to ensure that the therapist is knowledgeable about conducting exposure for anxiety. We say this because we firmly believe this treatment for illness anxiety is less likely to be helpful without significant practice in exposure to anxiety cues while refraining from excessive health behaviors. Therapists who conduct exposure therapy for anxiety disorders or obsessive-compulsive spectrum disorders are usually a good match.

A Final (but Very Important) Note

If you have read this far, congratulations on a really great job. Clearly, you are very persistent and motivated to work on your anxiety. If you have been practicing all the skills diligently, even better! You have really taken some difficult steps towards improving your life and talking back to the anxiety bully that follows us all around from time to time.

As you go forward living your valued life in pursuit of what you want, remember that improvement from anxiety issues and true mental health does not mean a lack of anxiety. Rather, it is having anxiety and *doing it anyway*. Living a valued life also does not mean a lack of physical symptoms, pain, discomfort, or uncertainty. It means acting on your values and living your life despite these things, not without them.

At its core, working on reducing illness anxiety is about tolerating uncertainty, and seeking less control over things. If you are like most people with illness anxiety, your health is likely not the only thing you want a high degree of control over. Our patients with health anxiety are often quite perfectionistic. They are typically highly intelligent, detail-oriented, successful high performers, but because of perfectionism and control desires, they are also people who have a very hard time tolerating situations when they are not in the driver's seat. It can be hard to acknowledge, but they often have some sense of arrogance, believing that they know more than most people, particularly about health, and cannot trust others to do as good a job as would meet their (often very high) standards. The illusion of control can be a powerful lure until you encounter situations that cannot be controlled, such as random health outcomes, and death and dying. If you continue to grasp at control and refrain from trying to trust educated others (i.e., doctors, loved ones) to make qualified decisions for you, you are losing out on opportunities to teach yourself that you can trust others and you are not alone in the world. If you are someone who wants a lot of control in several types of situations (and you probably are), we highly encourage you to gradually practice letting go of those control attempts and scientifically testing out your anxious feared outcomes just as you did with the exposures described in this book. What we are saying is that you do not need to restrain your practice in walking towards uncertainty and trusting others to the area of health anxiety, and we recommend you practice it in all areas of your life. As much as you are willing to practice this in your life, the more likely you are to neurobiologically teach your brain that not everything needs to be controlled, uncertainty is OK, and other people are trustworthy and intelligent.

Here's what we can guarantee you: for the rest of your life, you will continue to have intermittent unusual or uncomfortable physical sensations that surprise you. You will always have to live with the uncertainty that you *may* keel over at any minute, or at least some time soon. At some point in your life, you will be confronted with a legitimate medical concern, and if you are like most people, you will probably experience and survive several of them. Medical issues are part of life that all humans experience, and some level of anxiety about them is totally appropriate. Because these things happen, and because rare catastrophic outcomes could occur, does not mean that you must make your life overly cautious because of them. After all, if you regularly behaved in that way, you would never pursue relationships (they could leave you!), leave your home (bombs? shootings? natural disasters?), drive (accidents?), and so on. So we encourage you to welcome the uncertainty and walk out your door to a life that you want, leaving the illness anxiety ghost able to accompany you and talk at you, but never control you unless you want it to.

We feel privileged to have been able to walk you through the process of treatment, and grateful that you gave this book a read. We hope that you been able to get a good grounding in the treatment and have successfully worked through your therapeutic journey and seen significant decreases in your health anxiety. Hopefully, now you have a better understanding of how your health anxiety operates and the ways in which you can continue to address it successfully and feel better every day!

References

Chapter 1

1. Axelsson E, Hedman-Lagerlof E. Cognitive behavior therapy for health anxiety: systematic review and meta-analysis of clinical efficacy and health economic outcomes. *Expert Rev Pharmacoecon Outcomes Res.* 2019;19(6):663–676.
2. Norcross JC, Wampold BE. Evidence-based therapy relationships: Research conclusions and clinical practices. In: Norcross JC, ed. *Psychotherapy relationships that work: Evidence-based responsiveness.* 2nd ed. New York: Oxford University Press; 2011:423–430.
3. Lambert MJ, Barley DE. Research summary on the therapeutic relationship and psychotherapy outcome. *Psychotherapy.* 2001;38(4):357–361.
4. American Psychiatric Association. *Diagnostic and statistical manual of mental disorders.* 5th ed. Washington, DC: Author; 2013.
5. Reuman L, Jacoby RJ, Blakey SM, Riemann BC, Leonard RC, Abramowitz JS. Predictors of illness anxiety symptoms in patients with obsessive compulsive disorder. *Psychiatry Res.* 2017;256:417–422.
6. Bleichhardt G, Hiller W. Hypochondriasis and health anxiety in the German population. *Br J Health Psychol.* 2007;12(Pt 4):511–523.
7. Brakoulias V, Starcevic V, Belloch A, et al. Comorbidity, age of onset and suicidality in obsessive-compulsive disorder (OCD): An international collaboration. *Compr Psychiatry.* 2017;76:79–86.
8. Greeven A, van Balkom AJ, van Rood YR, van Oppen P, Spinhoven P. The boundary between hypochondriasis and obsessive-compulsive disorder: A cross-sectional study from the Netherlands. *J Clin Psychiatry.* 2006;67(11):1682–1689.
9. Pascual-Vera B, Belloch A. Dysmorphic and illness anxiety-related unwanted intrusive thoughts in individuals with obsessive-compulsive disorder. *Clin Psychol Psychother.* 2022;29(1):313–327.
10. Bailer J, Kerstner T, Witthoft M, Diener C, Mier D, Rist F. Health anxiety and hypochondriasis in the light of DSM-5. *Anxiety Stress Coping.* 2016;29(2):219–239.

11. Scarella TM, Boland RJ, Barsky AJ. Illness anxiety disorder: Psychopathology, epidemiology, clinical characteristics, and treatment. *Psychosom Med.* 2019;81(5):398–407.

12. Bandelow B, Reitt M, Rover C, Michaelis S, Gorlich Y, Wedekind D. Efficacy of treatments for anxiety disorders: A meta-analysis. *Int Clin Psychopharmacol.* 2015;30(4):183–192.

13. Carpenter JK, Andrews LA, Witcraft SM, Powers MB, Smits JAJ, Hofmann SG. Cognitive behavioral therapy for anxiety and related disorders: A meta-analysis of randomized placebo-controlled trials. *Depress Anxiety.* 2018;35(6):502–514.

14. Norton PJ, Price EC. A meta-analytic review of adult cognitive-behavioral treatment outcome across the anxiety disorders. *J Nerv Ment Dis.* 2007;195(6):521–531.

15. Butler AC, Chapman JE, Forman EM, Beck AT. The empirical status of cognitive-behavioral therapy: A review of meta-analyses. *Clin Psychol Rev.* 2006;26(1):17–31.

16. Olatunji BO, Kauffman BY, Meltzer S, Davis ML, Smits JA, Powers MB. Cognitive-behavioral therapy for hypochondriasis/health anxiety: A meta-analysis of treatment outcome and moderators. *Behav Res Ther.* 2014;58:65–74.

17. Fallon BA, Ahern DK, Pavlicova M, Slavov I, Skritskya N, Barsky AJ. A randomized controlled trial of medication and cognitive-behavioral therapy for hypochondriasis. *Am J Psychiatry.* 2017;174(8):756–764.

18. Hedman E, Axelsson E, Andersson E, Lekander M, Ljotsson B. Exposure-based cognitive-behavioural therapy via the internet and as bibliotherapy for somatic symptom disorder and illness anxiety disorder: Randomised controlled trial. *Br J Psychiatry.* 2016;209(5):407–413.

19. Hedman E, Andersson G, Andersson E, et al. Internet-based cognitive-behavioural therapy for severe health anxiety: Randomised controlled trial. *Br J Psychiatry.* 2011;198(3):230–236.

20. Fallon BA, Liebowitz MR, Salman E, et al. Fluoxetine for hypochondriacal patients without major depression. *J Clin Psychopharmacol.* 1993;13(6):438–441.

21. Greeven A, van Balkom AJ, Visser S, et al. Cognitive behavior therapy and paroxetine in the treatment of hypochondriasis: A randomized controlled trial. *Am J Psychiatry.* 2007;164(1):91–99.

22. Fineberg NA, Pellegrini L, Clarke A, et al. Meta-analysis of cognitive behaviour therapy and selective serotonin reuptake inhibitors for the treatment of hypochondriasis: Implications for trial design. *Compr Psychiatry.* 2022;118:152334.
23. Schweitzer PJ, Zafar U, Pavlicova M, Fallon BA. Long-term follow-up of hypochondriasis after selective serotonin reuptake inhibitor treatment. *J Clin Psychopharmacol.* 2011;31(3):365–368.
24. Baldwin DS, Anderson IM, Nutt DJ, et al. Evidence-based pharmacological treatment of anxiety disorders, post-traumatic stress disorder and obsessive-compulsive disorder: A revision of the 2005 guidelines from the British Association for Psychopharmacology. *J Psychopharmacol.* 2014;28(5):403–439.
25. Baldwin DS, Anderson IM, Nutt DJ, et al. Evidence-based guidelines for the pharmacological treatment of anxiety disorders: Recommendations from the British Association for psychopharmacology. *J Psychopharmacol.* 2005;19(6):567–596.
26. Katzman MA, Bleau P, Blier P, et al. Canadian clinical practice guidelines for the management of anxiety, posttraumatic stress and obsessive-compulsive disorders. *BMC Psychiatry.* 2014;14(Suppl 1):S1.
27. Andrews G, Bell C, Wilkins G. Royal australian and New Zealand College of psychiatrists clinical practice guidelines for panic disorder, social anxiety disorder, and generalised anxiety disorder. *Aust. N. Z. J. Psychiatry.* 2018;52(12):1109–1172.
28. Wetherell JL, Petkus AJ, White KS, et al. Antidepressant medication augmented with cognitive-behavioral therapy for generalized anxiety disorder in older adults. *Am J Psychiatry.* 2013;170(7):782–789.
29. Abramowitz J, Deacon B, Whiteside S. *Exposure therapy for anxiety: Principles and practice.* New York: Guilford Press; 2019.
30. Hofmann SG, Sawyer AT, Korte KJ, Smits JAJ. Is it beneficial to add pharmacotherapy to cognitive-behavioral therapy when treating anxiety disorders? A meta-analytic review. *International Journal of Cognitive Therapy.* 2009;2(2):160–175.
31. Manthey L, van Veen T, Giltay EJ, et al. Correlates of (inappropriate) benzodiazepine use: The Netherlands Study of Depression and Anxiety (NESDA). *Br J Clin Pharmacol.* 2011;71(2):263–272.
32. Bandelow B, Michaelis S, Wedekind D. Treatment of anxiety disorders. *Dialogues Clin Neurosci.* 2017;19(2):93–107.

33. Agarwal SD, Landon BE. Patterns in outpatient benzodiazepine prescribing in the United States. *JAMA Netw Open.* 2019;2(1):e187399.

34. Guina J, Merrill B. Benzodiazepines I: Upping the care on downers: The evidence of risks, benefits and alternatives. *J Clin Med.* 2018;7(2):17.

35. Westra HA, Stewart SH, Conrad BE. Naturalistic manner of benzodiazepine use and cognitive behavioral therapy outcome in panic disorder with agoraphobia. *J Anxiety Disord.* 2002;16(3):233–246.

36. Otto MW, Pollack MH, Sabatino SA. Maintenance of remission following cognitive-behavior therapy for panic disorder: Possible deleterious effects of concurrent medication treatment. *Behav Ther.* 1996;27:473–482.

37. Salkovskis PM, Rimes KA, Warwick HM, Clark DM. The health anxiety inventory: Development and validation of scales for the measurement of health anxiety and hypochondriasis. *Psychol Med.* 2002;32(5):843–853.

38. Escobar JI, Gara M, Waitzkin H, Silver RC, Holman A, Compton W. DSM-IV hypochondriasis in primary care. *Gen Hosp Psychiatry.* 1998;20(3):155–159.

39. Weck F, Richtberg S, Neng JM. Epidemilogy of hypochondriasis and health anxiety: Comparison of different diagnostic criteria. *Curr Psychiatry Rev.* 2010;10:14–23.

40. Dunn D, Donato S, Keenan-Miller D. Perceived helpfulness of previous therapy: A predictor of premature termination. *Prof Psychol Res Pract.* 2023;54(4):275–283.

41. Bobevski I, Clarke DM, Meadows G. Health anxiety and its relationship to disability and service use: Findings from a large epidemiological survey. *Psychosom Med.* 2016;78(1):13–25.

42. Seivewright H, Salkovskis P, Green J, et al. Prevalence and service implications of health anxiety in genitourinary medicine clinics. *Int J STD AIDS.* 2004;15(8):519–522.

43. Sunderland M, Newby JM, Andrews G. Health anxiety in Australia: Prevalence, comorbidity, disability and service use. *Br J Psychiatry.* 2013;202(1):56–61.

44. Fink P, Ornbol E, Christensen KS. The outcome of health anxiety in primary care. A two-year follow-up study on health care costs and self-rated health. *PLoS One.* 2010;5(3):e9873.

45. Barsky AJ, Fama JM, Bailey ED, Ahern DK. A prospective 4- to 5-year study of DSM-III-R hypochondriasis. *Arch Gen Psychiatry.* 1998;55(8):737–744.
46. Eilenberg T, Frostholm L, Schroder A, Jensen JS, Fink P. Long-term consequences of severe health anxiety on sick leave in treated and untreated patients: Analysis alongside a randomised controlled trial. *J Anxiety Disord.* 2015;32:95–102.

Chapter 2

1. Park J, Moghaddam B. Impact of anxiety on prefrontal cortex encoding of cognitive flexibility. *Neuroscience.* 2017;345:193–202.
2. Park J, Wood J, Bondi C, Del Arco A, Moghaddam B. Anxiety evokes hypofrontality and disrupts rule-relevant encoding by dorsomedial prefrontal cortex neurons. *J Neurosci.* 2016;36(11):3322–3335.
3. Bishop S, Duncan J, Brett M, Lawrence AD. Prefrontal cortical function and anxiety: Controlling attention to threat-related stimuli. *Nat Neurosci.* 2004;7(2):184–188.
4. Reuman L, Jacoby RJ, Blakey SM, Riemann BC, Leonard RC, Abramowitz JS. Predictors of illness anxiety symptoms in patients with obsessive compulsive disorder. *Psychiatry Res.* 2017;256:417–422.
5. Arnaez S, Garcia-Soriano G, Lopez-Santiago J, Belloch A. Dysfunctional beliefs as mediators between illness-related intrusive thoughts and health anxiety symptoms. *Behav Cogn Psychother.* 2020;48(3):315–326.
6. Gellatly R, Beck AT. Catastrophic thinking: A transdiagnostic process across psychiatric disorders. *Cognitive Therapy and Research.* 2016;40:441–452.
7. Marcus DK, Hughes KT, Arnau RC. Health anxiety, rumination, and negative affect: A mediational analysis. *J Psychosom Res.* 2008;64(5):495–501.
8. Owens KMB, Admunsdon GJG, Hadjistavropoulos T, Owens T. Attentional biase toward illness threat in individuals with elevated health anxiety. *Cognitive Therapy and Research.* 2004;28(1):57–66.
9. Barsky AJ, Wyshak G, Klerman GL. The somatosensory amplification scale and its relationship to hypochondriasis. *J Psychiatr Res.* 1990;24(4):323–334.

10. Grossi D, Longarzo M, Quarantelli M, et al. Altered functional connectivity of interoception in illness anxiety disorder. *Cortex*. 2017;86:22–32.

11. Hansen KF. Approaching doomsday: How SARS was presented in the Norwegian media. *Journal of Risk Research*. 2009(3–4): 345–360.

12. Albery IP, Spada MM, Nikcevic AV. The COVID-19 anxiety syndrome and selective attentional bias towards COVID-19-related stimuli in UK residents during the 2020-2021 pandemic. *Clin Psychol Psychother*. 2021;28(6):1367–1378.

13. Stefan S, Zorila A, Brie E. General threat and health-related attention biases in illness anxiety disorder: A brief research report. *Cognition & Emotion*. 2020;34(3):604–613.

14. Lees A, Mogg K, Bradley BP. Health anxiety, anxiety sensitivity, and attentional biases for pictorial and linguistic health-threat cues. *Cogn Emot*. 2005;19(3):453–462.

15. Owens M, Harrison AJ, Burkhouse KL, et al. Eye tracking indices of attentional bias in children of depressed mothers: Polygenic influences help to clarify previous mixed findings. *Dev Psychopathol*. 2016;28(2):385–397.

16. Shi C, Taylor S, Witthoft M, et al. Attentional bias toward health-threat in health anxiety: A systematic review and three-level meta-analysis. *Psychol Med*. 2022;52(4):604–613.

17. Feigin VL, Nguyen G, Cercy KBS, et al. Global, regional, and country-specific lifetime risks of stroke, 1990 and 2016. *N Engl J Med*. 2018;379:2429–2437.

18. National Safety Council. NSC Injury Facts: Preventable Deaths. 2022; https://injuryfacts.nsc.org/all-injuries/preventable-death-overview/odds-of-dying/. Accessed 06/23/2022.

19. National Weather Service. How Dangerous is Lightening? 2023; https://www.weather.gov/safety/lightning-odds. Accessed 09/22/2023.

20. Center for Disease Control and Prevention. Venemous Snakes. 2021; https://www.cdc.gov/niosh/topics/snakes/default.html. Accessed 09/11/2023, 2023.

21. Ma L, Danoff TM, Borish L. Case fatality and population mortality associated with anaphylaxis in the united states. *J Allergy Clin Immunol.* 2014;133:1075–1083.

Chapter 3

1. Wegner DM, Schneider DJ, Carter SR, White TL. Paradoxical effects of thought suppression. *J. Pers. Soc. Psychol.* 1987;53:5–13.

Chapter 4

1. Barsky AJ, Wyshak G, Klerman GL. The somatosensory amplification scale and its relationship to hypochondriasis. *J Psychiatr Res.* 1990;24(4):323–334.
2. Grossi D, Longarzo M, Quarantelli M, et al. Altered functional connectivity of interoception in illness anxiety disorder. *Cortex.* 2017;86:22–32.
3. Berdy J. Thoughts and facts about antibiotics: Where we are now and where we are heading. *J Antibiot (Tokyo).* 2012;65(8):441.
4. Shallcross LJ, Davies DS. GP antibiotic overuse and microbial resistance. *Br J Gen Pract.* 2015;65(631):61–62.
5. Centers for Disease Control and Prevention. Leading Causes of Death. *FastStats Homepage* 2023; https://www.cdc.gov/nchs/fastats/leading-causes-of-death.htm. Accessed 10/02/2023.
6. Martin A, Jacobi F. Features of hypochondriasis and illness worry in the general population in Germany. *Psychosom Med.* 2006;68(5):770–777.
7. Hollifield M, Paine S, Tuttle L, Kellner R. Hypochondriasis, somatization, and perceived health and utilization of health care services. *Psychosomatics.* 1999;40(5):380–386.
8. Barsky AJ, Wyshak G, Klerman GL. Hypochondriasis. An evaluation of the DSM-III criteria in medical outpatients. *Arch Gen Psychiatry.* 1986;43(5):493–500.
9. Barsky AJ, Fama JM, Bailey ED, Ahern DK. A prospective 4- to 5-year study of DSM-III-R hypochondriasis. *Arch Gen Psychiatry.* 1998;55(8):737–744.

10. Brownlee S, Chalkidou K, Doust J, et al. Evidence for overuse of medical services around the world. *Lancet.* 2017;390(10090):156–168.
11. Hurley R. Can doctors reduce harmful medical overuse worldwide? *BMJ.* 2014;349:g4289.
12. Schwind J, Neng JM, Hofling V, Weck F. Health behavior in hypochondriasis. *J Nerv Ment Dis.* 2015;203(7):493–498.

Chapter 5

1. Axelsson E, Hedman-Lagerlof E. Cognitive behavior therapy for health anxiety: Systematic review and meta-analysis of clinical efficacy and health economic outcomes. *Expert Rev Pharmacoecon Outcomes Res.* 2019;19(6):663–676.
2. Deacon BJ, Abramowitz JS. Cognitive and behavioral treatments for anxiety disorders: A review of meta-analytic findings. *J Clin Psychol.* 2004;60(4):429–441.
3. McLean CP, Levy HC, Miller ML, Tolin DF. Exposure therapy for PTSD: A meta-analysis. *Clin Psychol Rev.* 2022;91:102115.
4. Weck F, Neng JM, Richtberg S, Jakob M, Stangier U. Cognitive therapy versus exposure therapy for hypochondriasis (health anxiety): A randomized controlled trial. *J Consult Clin Psychol.* 2015;83(4):665–676.
5. Ferrando C, Selai C. A systematic review and meta-analysis on the effectiveness of exposure and response prevention therapy in the treatment of obsessive-compulsive disorder. *J Obsessive Compul Relat Disord.* 2021;31:100684.
6. Gallagher MW, Payne LA, White KS, et al. Mechanisms of change in cognitive behavioral therapy for panic disorder: The unique effects of self-efficacy and anxiety sensitivity. *Behav Res Ther.* 2013;51(11):767–777.
7. Goldin PR, Ziv M, Jazaieri H, et al. Cognitive reappraisal self-efficacy mediates the effects of individual cognitive-behavioral therapy for social anxiety disorder. *J. Consult. Clin. Psychol.* 2012;80(6):1034–1040.
8. Craske MG, Kircanski K, Zelikowsky M, Mystkowski J, Chowdhury N, Baker A. Optimizing inhibitory learning during exposure therapy. *Behav Res Ther.* 2008;46(1):5–27.

9. Jungmann SM, Witthoft M. Health anxiety, cyberchondria, and coping in the current COVID-19 pandemic: Which factors are related to coronavirus anxiety? *J Anxiety Disord*. 2020;73:102239.
10. Te Poel F, Baumgartner SE, Hartmann T, Tanis M. The curious case of cyberchondria: A longitudinal study on the reciprocal relationship between health anxiety and online health information seeking. *J Anxiety Disord*. 2016;43:32–40.
11. Brown RJ, Skelly N, Chew-Graham CA. Online health research and health anxiety: A systematic review and conceptual integration. *Clin Psychol Sci Pract*. 2018;27(2):1–19.

Chapter 6

1. Fergus TA, Valentiner DP. Disease phobia and disease conviction are separate dimensions underlying hypochondriasis. *J Behav Ther Exp Psychiatry*. 2010;41(4):438–444.

Chapter 7

1. Lickel J, Nelson E, Hayes AH, Deacon B. Interoceptive exposure exercises for evoking depersonalization and derealization: A pilot study. *J Cogn Psychother*. 2008;22(4):321–330.

Chapter 8

1. Goldman N, Dugas MJ, Sexton KA, Gervais NJ. The impact of written exposure on worry: a preliminary investigation. *Behav Modif*. 2007;31(4):512–538.
2. Kaplan J, Tolin D. Exposure therapy for anxiety disorders: Theoretical mechanisms of exposure and treatment strategies. *Psychiatr Times*. 2011;28(9):9.
3. Bryant RA, Moulds ML, Guthrie RM, Dang ST, Nixon RD. Imaginal exposure alone and imaginal exposure with cognitive restructuring in treatment of posttraumatic stress disorder. *J Consult Clin Psychol*. 2003;71(4):706–712.

4. Foa EB, Steketee G, Turner RM, Fischer SC. Effects of imaginal exposure to feared disasters in obsessive-compulsive checkers. *Behav Res Ther.* 1980;18(5):449–455.
5. Pew Research Center. The global religious landscape. *Religious Demographics.* 2012; https://www.pewresearch.org/religion/2012/12/18/global-religious-landscape-exec/.
6. Shreve-Neiger AK, Edelstein BA. Religion and anxiety: a critical review of the literature. *Clin Psychol Rev.* 2004;24(4):379–397.

Chapter 9

1. Gao J, Zheng P, Jia Y, et al. Mental health problems and social media exposure during COVID-19 outbreak. *PLoS One.* 2020;15(4):e0231924.
2. Roy D, Tripathy S, Kar SK, Sharma N, Verma SK, Kaushal V. Study of knowledge, attitude, anxiety & perceived mental healthcare need in Indian population during COVID-19 pandemic. *Asian J Psychiatr.* 2020;51:102083.

Chapter 10

1. Aldao A, Nolen-Hoeksema S, Schweizer S. Emotion-regulation strategies across psychopathology: A meta-analytic review. *Clin Psychol Rev.* 2010;30(2):217–237.
2. Amstadter A. Emotion regulation and anxiety disorders. *J Anxiety Disord.* 2008;22:211–221.
3. Mattingley S, Youssef GJ, Manning V, Graeme L, Hall K. Distress tolerance across substance use, eating, and borderline personality disorders: A meta-analysis. *J Affect Disord.* 2022;300:492–504.
4. McHugh RK, Kertz SJ, Weiss RB, Baskin-Sommers AR, Hearon BA, Bjorgvinsson T. Changes in distress intolerance and treatment outcome in a partial hospital setting. *Behav Ther.* 2014;45(2):232–240.
5. Simons JS, Simons RM, Grimm KJ, Keith JA, Stoltenberg SF. Affective dynamics among veterans: Associations with distress tolerance and posttraumatic stress symptoms. *Emotion.* 2021;21(4):757–771.
6. Zhong J, Huang XJ, Wang XM, Xu MZ. The mediating effect of distress tolerance on the relationship between stressful life events

and suicide risk in patients with major depressive disorder. *BMC Psychiatry*. 2023;23(1):118.

7. Bernstein A, Marshall EC, Zvolensky M. Multi-method evaluation of distress tolerance measures and construct(s): Concurrent relations to mood and anxiety psychopathology and quality of life. *J Exp Psychopathol*. 2011;2(3):386–399.

8. Yardley P, McCall A, Savage A, Newton R. Effectiveness of a brief intervention aimed at increasing distress tolerance for individuals in crisis or at risk of self-harm. *Australas Psychiatry*. 2019;27(6):565–568.

9. Bornovalova MA, Gratz KL, Daughters SB, Hunt ED, Lejuez CW. Initial RCT of a distress tolerance treatment for individuals with substance use disorders. *Drug Alcohol Depend*. 2012;122(1–2):70–76.

10. Heiland AM, Veilleux JC. Reductions in distress intolerance via intervention: A review. *Cogn Behav Ther*. 2023. https://psycnet.apa .org/doi/10.1007/s10608-023-10425-1.

11. Sauer KS, Witthoft M. Inhibitory learning versus habituation in an experimental exposure intervention for people with heightened health anxiety: Increase of distress tolerance as a joint mechanism of change? *Journal of experimental psychopathology*. 2022(October–December);13(4):204380872211387.

12. Gallagher MW, Payne LA, White KS, et al. Mechanisms of change in cognitive behavioral therapy for panic disorder: The unique effects of self-efficacy and anxiety sensitivity. *Behav Res Ther*. 2013;51(11):767–777.

13. Song S, Yang X, Yang H, et al. Psychological resilience as a protective factor for depression and anxiety among the public during the outbreak of COVID-19. *Front Psychol*. 2021;11. https://doi.org/10.3389/fpsyg.2020.618509.

14. Nolen-Hoeksema S. The role of rumination in depressive disorders and mixed anxiety/depressive symptoms. *J Abnorm Psychol*. 2000;109(3):504–511.

15. Cloninger CR, Zohar AH, Hirschmann S, Dahan D. The psychological costs and benefits of being highly persistent: Personality profiles distinguish mood disorders from anxiety disorders. *J Affect Disord*. 2012;136(3):758–766.

Chapter 11

1. Salkovskis PM, Rimes KA, Warwick HM, Clark DM. The health anxiety inventory: Development and validation of scales for the measurement of health anxiety and hypochondriasis. *Psychol Med.* 2002;32(5):843–853.
2. Baier AL, Kline AC, Feeny NC. Therapeutic alliance as a mediator of change: A systematic review and evaluation of research. *Clin Psychol Rev.* 2020;82:101921.
3. Martin DJ, Garske JP, Davis MK. Relation of the therapeutic alliance with outcome and other variables: A meta-analytic review. *J Consult Clin Psychol.* 2000;68(3):438–450.

Index

agoraphobia 12
antidepressant medication 18–19

benzodiazepines 19

catastrophizing 48–50
cognitive-behavioral treatment 16
cognitive distortions 136
cyberchondria 112

depersonalization *see* derealization
derealization 166
downward arrow 40–41

ego-dystonic thoughts 8
ego-syntonic 248
emotional reasoning 140
exposure: description of 98; rationale for use 99–102

fortune telling (cognitive distortion) 139

Generalized anxiety disorder (GAD) 13

health anxiety inventory-short version 22, 255
health anxiety *see* illness anxiety disorder
hypochondriasis 6; *see also* illness anxiety disorder

illness anxiety disorder: definition 2; diagnosis 5–6; prevalence 7
imaginal exposures: description 190; examples 195–199; rationale 190–195
interoceptive exposures: description 153, 157; examples 158–166, 176–178; rationale 153–155

labeling (cognitive distortion) 140

magical thinking 86–87, 96–97; related exposures 114
magnification 137–138
mind reading (cognitive distortion) 127

obsessive-compulsive disorder 7

panic disorder 11
post-traumatic stress disorder 14

relapse prevention 254–255, 259

safety behaviors 121
self-monitoring 34
Should statements (cognitive distortion) 141
somatic symptom disorder 10
SSRI medications 19
Subjective Units of Distress Scale (SUDS) 108–109

thought-action fusion 86

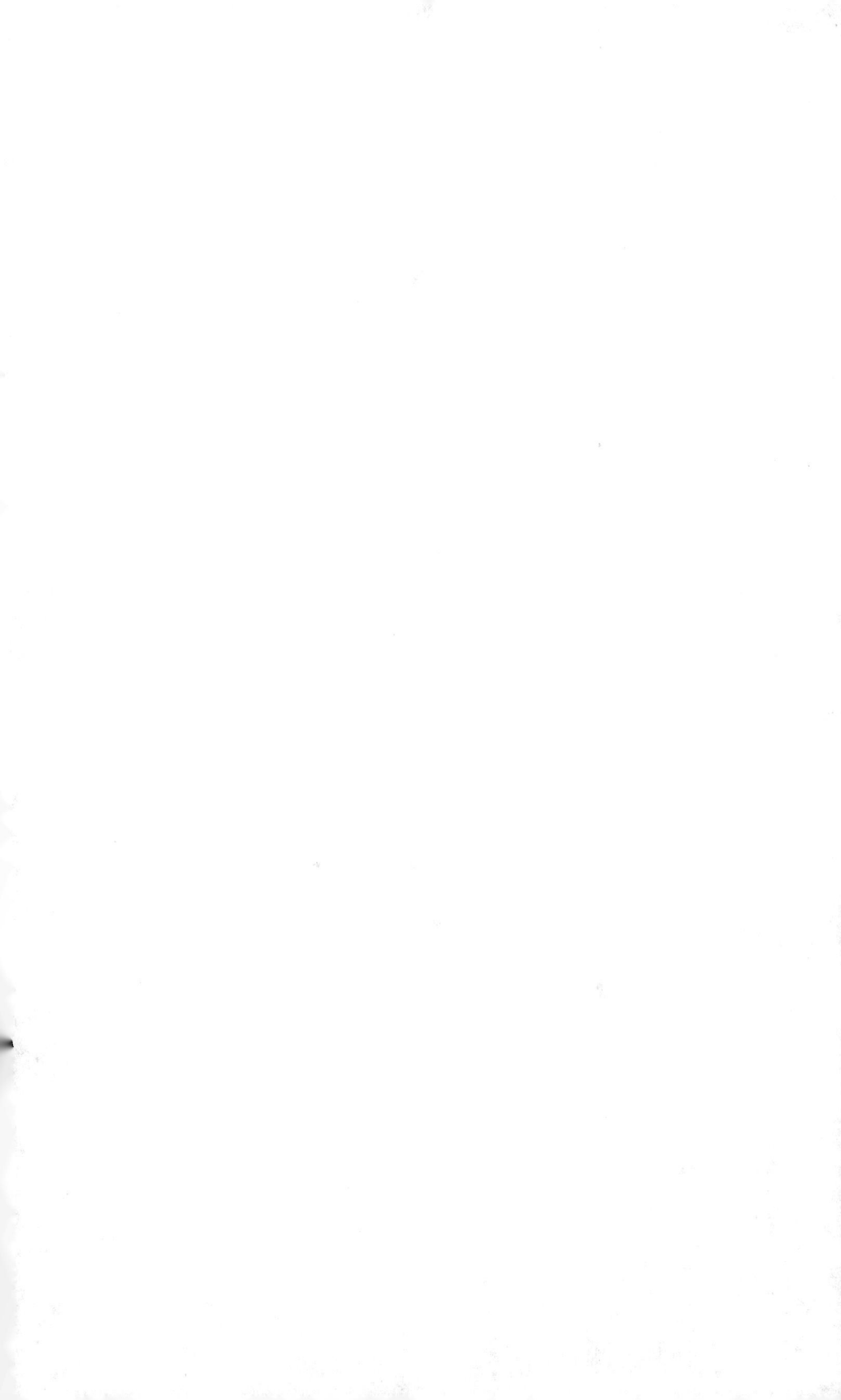

For Product Safety Concerns and Information please contact our EU
representative GPSR@taylorandfrancis.com
Taylor & Francis Verlag GmbH, Kaufingerstraße 24, 80331 München, Germany